Banish Post-baby Blues

BANISH
POST-BABY BLUES

All the advice, support and encouragement you
need to cope with post-natal depression

Anne-Marie Sapsted

THORSONS PUBLISHING GROUP

First published in 1990

British Library Cataloguing in Publication Data

Sapsted, Anne-Marie
Banish post-baby blues.
1. Women. Post natal depression
I. Title
618.76

ISBN 0-7225-2123-5

*Published by Thorsons Publishing Group,
Wellingborough, Northamptonshire NN8 2RQ, England*

Typeset by Harper Phototypesetters Limited, Northampton
Printed in Great Britain by Mackays of Chatham, Kent

3 5 7 9 10 8 6 4 2

Contents

Acknowledgements

There are a number of people I must thank who were helpful and supportive in the preparation of this book.

Firstly, thanks to Vivienne Parry, national organiser of Birthright, the mother and baby charity, who invited me to a conference on post-natal depression which was my starting point. Thanks to my own health visitor who put me in touch with several women she had contact with who were suffering from the illness. Thanks to Virginia Ironside, agony aunt on the *Sunday Mirror*, a good friend and advisor. Thanks to Kate Allen, the editor of the book, who made it work.

But most of all, thanks to all the women who were prepared to talk to me about the pain and suffering that is post-natal depression.

Foreword

Mental illness is a surprisingly common complication following childbirth. Although maternal morality and rates of complications of delivery have fallen dramatically in the last fifty years, there seems to be little change in the rates of mental illness. Post-natal depression alone probably occurs in 10 per cent of births, and the months following birth of the first child are the time at which a woman is most vulnerable to mental illness. There is still too little known about post-natal mental illness although there has been some increase in both medical and research knowledge and awareness among the general public. There is still a need for not only a readable account but also some constructive suggestions about what can be done to help and this book fills both these needs.

Anne-Marie Sapsted describes vividly, with a journalist's perceptive eye, the experience of post-natal mental illness. She has also read very widely and become familiar with the psychological and psychiatric background and recent research progress.

The book will take the reader through the types of post-natal illness, and the 'blues' of the title are placed in context. There is no attempt to avoid contentious issues (e.g. the real incidence of post-natal depression; the power of hormones; the influence of medical technology).

Fathers too rarely get more than a mention in books about childbirth and yet we know how important social support is at other times of stress. Many bewildered partners will find help here. There is no repetition of accepted wisdom but the courage to question (e.g. do fathers *have* to be present at the moment of birth?).

Psychologists are becoming more and more aware of the importance of the concept of self-esteem and a woman's self-esteem is never more threatened than when she first becomes a mother. Many women try too hard to become supermums and are inevitably going to feel failures. How reassuring to a working mother to find that someone else understands about guilt. Vivid personal accounts make this a hard book to put down. If you want to get some insight into the meaning and experience of post-natal mental illness or if you haven't talked to someone about PND these descriptions will give great insight. If you have, you will recognize their desperate plight.

This is not just another account of the struggle of parenthood. There is no fruitless searching for causes or laying the blame entirely on hospitals, hormones or life events. Many of us who work in the field suspect that the psychiatric diagnosis of PND is the tip of the iceberg and many mothers experience depressive symptoms that might not rate 'caseness', yet are none the less very distressing.

Anne-Marie Sapsted gives constructive help which has been lacking in previous books. From the Action Plan to Sources of Help, there is a large section on what a mother can do to help herself or for others to help her.

I hope that fewer and fewer mothers will be able to say 'nobody helps you to understand the complexity of emotions that come with childbirth' (Carmen's story). There are many concerned clinicians and health professionals and a number of research endeavours in the field. One of the difficulties is that the problems of post-natal depression cross many disciplines. The Marcé Society is an international multi-disciplinary society which aims to improve knowledge about post-natal mental illness and to disseminate information to professionals and the general public. Anne-Marie Sapsted has made a valuable contribution to these aims.

This remarkable book will provide insight, comfort and practical help and no one reading it could remain unconvinced of the distress of post-natal depression and they will also see that with help, 'blues' can be banished.

Elizabeth Alder Ph.D., C.Psychol.
Lecturer in Psychology, Queen Margaret College, Edinburgh
and Secretary of the Marcé Society

Preface

Very little has been written for women suffering from post-natal depression (PND). When I was researching this book, many sufferers said that they wished they could have talked to, or at least read about, others with similar experiences, as it would have helped to know that they were not suffering alone. For this reason I have included several detailed case histories.

In my search for these case histories, I was expecting to have to undertake a lengthy process of research to find people prepared to come forward and tell me about their experiences. It is a measure of just how widespread post-natal depression is that all I had to do was mention it to friends and colleagues and every one of them, it seemed, knew about it. Either they had suffered themselves to some degree — often to my surprise — or they knew someone who had suffered. I also made contact, via the health services, with several mothers who either were suffering or had suffered from PND. In no time at all, I had a large group of women who were happy to talk to me in detail about their experience.

It seems to me that while each case is different, there are also threads common to them all. Two of these stand out: firstly, the way victims of this illness fail to come to the attention of not only their doctors, midwives and health visitors, but also their own families. Secondly, without exception, what these women needed most was to talk to someone who understood exactly what they were going through. For the few who did receive help from professionals, it is notable that this help was seldom available and, even when it was, often inappropriate. It is also notable that the diagnosis of post-natal depression was often made when the illness was over, when the victim had recovered.

Depression after giving birth is a particularly cruel illness, it seems to me, in that most sufferers blame themselves for the way they are feeling. They focus on what they see as their own inadequacies and inabilities to cope. They think of themselves as 'bad mothers'. Time and again in the course of writing this book I was told how the image of the 'Perfect Mother and Baby' as portrayed on television and in magazines was one they struggled to live up to — and saw themselves as failing at. Sufferers from PND see themselves surrounded by happy women basking in the glow of motherhood. After all, they have been told so many times: 'Aren't you lucky having such a lovely baby? You must be very happy!'

When talking to another journalist who had also tackled this subject while living in America, I was told that she had been amazed to discover that in some parts of the USA post-natal depression is scarcely recognized as an illness. After talking about it on American radio and television, she was inundated with calls from women asking for her help in the face of an apparent lack of interest from their doctors. In Australia and New Zealand it seems things are a little better, with a growing network of self-help and support groups. In Britain, too, the picture is slowly changing. Gradually we are coming to accept that the illness called post-natal depression is not only about those very few women who are so ill they are driven to suicide and even to killing their own children, but also about the thousands of mothers who are more often than not suffering in silence.

CHAPTER ONE
The myth of the perfect birth

Few women seem to be aware that depression is the most common complication following childbirth. In fact, many women are not aware of the existence of post-natal depression at all. Of the millions of live births every year worldwide — 750,000 in the UK alone — it is estimated that around one in ten of all new mothers will become depressed. That figure stays the same year after year. Yet over the last 50 years or so enormous effort has been put into reducing the maternal mortality rate, and with great success, so that now only 0.1 per cent of mothers die in childbirth. Add to that the fact that another 95 per cent of all deliveries in the Western world take place in hospitals where women are surrounded by every modern diagnostic tool as well as by highly trained, specialized staff. Figures for PND, however, still have not changed.

There are a number of other significant statistics which should also be considered:

- Of the 1 in 10 mothers who become depressed, only 1 in 100 are ever seen by a psychiatrist and over 50 are not seen by anyone at all.

- A large number of the women who do complain about feeling depressed are simply handed tranquillizers by their doctors, a remedy which is often completely inappropriate.

- The first-time mother has a 35-times greater chance of being referred to a psychiatrist than at any other time in her life.

- If women suffer from post-natal depression after their first baby, a second pregnancy increases the chances of its recurrence. Experts vary on the likelihood or recurrence but estimates suggest anywhere between 20-70 per cent.

● 2 out of every 5 depressed mothers go on to suffer other periods of depression within four years.

● Women are 16 times more likely to have a psychiatric illness of some kind in the first three months after childbirth than at any other time in their lives.

● For many women, childbirth is the beginning of life-long psychiatric illness.

What is post-natal depression?

Post-natal depression lies somewhere in the middle of a band of conditions labelled post-natal illness. At one end lies the very common 'blues' and at the other the very severe, and fortunately rare, puerperal psychosis.

Most women have heard of the 'post-baby blues' and most women suffer from these blues in the first few days after the birth. This is a time when they feel very emotional and find themselves bursting into tears for apparently no reason. A woman cannot explain why she feels like this and cannot be jollied out of it. This feeling doesn't usually last longer than a couple of days and is the one form of depression which most women are warned about, either by friends or professionals. It is ironic, considering its relative unimportance, that it is also the form which most people seem willing to accept and be sympathetic about.

It has been suggested by some that this form of post-natal depression is associated with the rapidly changing hormonal levels in the body which are occurring naturally in the first few days after the birth. It has also been linked to the normal weight loss experienced by most women at this time.

Puerperal psychosis is at the opposite end of the spectrum of post-natal illness. It is severe, but fortunately rare. The sufferer becomes unable to function normally with either manic or depressive symptoms which no one can ignore. Admission to a psychiatric hospital is almost always the only way of treating this condition, but sufferers usually react quickly and well to treatment and make a complete recovery.

Manic symptoms include very pronounced euphoria and excitement. The mother cannot stop talking, speaks very quickly in broken sentences and the ideas expressed are difficult to understand. She seems able to keep going without sleep and often cannot find the time to eat. She gradually loses her sense of reality, and may become destructive and aggressive if anyone disagrees with her.

Depressive symptoms include an inability to smile or laugh about anything. The mother may spend the whole day in tears, and gradually becomes more and more unable to cope with even the simplest task or decision about everyday life. She may suffer panic attacks, is unable to relax, and is eventually completely unable to care for her baby. She cannot concentrate and often becomes obsessional. Many normal functions are impaired, such as sleeping and eating.

Treatments include anti-depressant drugs (these are not addictive); hormone therapy; electroconvulsive therapy (ECT), a controversial treatment which involves passing an electric current through the brain to produce a convulsion, and which can sometimes be very effective, very quickly; or psycho-therapy, group therapy or some other form of 'talking' therapy.

In speaking to women who suffer from PND, it is particularly striking how many suffer in silence for sometimes months on end. In the majority of cases they keep their feelings locked in, even denying to themselves that anything is wrong. Women who are very sick somehow manage to convince husbands and family that they are coping. The following two case histories graphically illustrate the seriousness of the condition. In some ways the two stories are quite different: for example, the women come from opposite ends of the social scale. But there are striking similarities. Both somehow managed to keep on running a home and neither was taken seriously by those around her.

Both women were eventually told that they had suffered from post-natal depression, but because of the lack of adequate treatment, both continue to suffer in some way. Neither will say that they have completely recovered and will admit to suffering bouts of general depression, or just 'feeling down' from time to time, in a way that they did not feel before they fell victim to PND. It is important to emphasize, though, that neither woman sought or received the best help available — help which can bring about a complete recovery.

Margaret's story

I think my problem started a couple of months before my second baby was born. I woke up one morning and just didn't want to do anything. I couldn't cope with the kids or the house. I hated myself. I was going through a divorce at the time and I felt really desperate. I went to the doctor, got some help and began to feel a bit better, but I've continued to suffer from depression ever since.

I didn't have much of a happy childhood myself and like most new mums I had no experience with babies. They go on in books and on TV about how it's all lovely, how having babies will bring you and your partner closer together. But it's not like that. I'm 20 and I've been married for four years. We'd been married for just over a year when I had the first baby and he was only 18 months old when I was pregnant again — another boy. It was all very quick. When the youngest was about a year old, I started to feel really down again. I felt very, very down. The baby was very quiet but I just couldn't cope with him — in fact I was only giving him a little bit to eat, starving him, although I didn't mean to. The health visitor noticed he was a bit underweight and then I told her how I was feeling and she arranged for me to see the GP and he sent me to see a psychiatrist.

The psychiatrist just kept asking the same questions over and over again, repeating everything I said. It was like being interrogated. He wasn't sympathetic at all. At home I was having more and more rows with my husband. He couldn't have cared less about anything. He thought I was nuts. My family were no help. They accused me of doing all this to get attention. They all said I was a terrible mother. They told me to pull myself together. I got no support.

Eventually, the children went to stay with their grandparents. I kept asking myself: 'Am I a good mother?' I didn't have many friends and I didn't let my feelings out to anyone. I used to drive around in the car like a lunatic just looking for someone to talk to. My parents didn't want to know.

In the end it all got too much and I got suicidal and took some tablets. The health visitor came round just after I'd taken them and said I'd got to go to hospital. I can't remember much after I got there. I just didn't want to wake up.

My husband didn't even come to see me when I was in the hospital. When I got home he was even more nasty. The doctor was no help either. He gave me tablets and they just made me sleepy. They give you tablets and then just talk to you as if there's nothing really wrong. I went up to the surgery in tears but it didn't make any difference. I think he should have been a bit more understanding.

Then my mother tried to keep the children. She'd got very fond of them while looking after them, and she wouldn't let me have them back. I went straight up to see the doctor, and he was a help then. He told me I would get them back.

A psychiatric nurse used to come to the house. I couldn't stand that. He couldn't understand what I was trying to say. They don't seem to understand what is happening in these cases. I didn't find him any help at all. We tried marriage guidance for a while, but all it was was my husband saying: 'You were terrible, you were horrible,' as if it was just me like it. I can't talk to him about any problems. I just get further and further down. I feel he's pulling me down. He picks an argument when I'm down in the dumps. A friend of mine who's had a baby has just got post-natal depression, but her husband is really sympathetic and he's helping her through. Husbands are the ones who should notice things going wrong and do something about it. My husband must have noticed that I wasn't right, that I wasn't getting up, and that kind of thing. But . . . he finds it hard to cope with illness.

Well, I've decided it's not going to get the better of me. Now I sit myself down with a cup of tea and a fag until I feel better and then I make myself do things. Gradually every day I do a bit more. I used to have to go out all the time. I couldn't stand to be here on my own, but that's a bit better now.

When I was a teenager I suffered from depression because of what was going on at home. My parents used to argue a lot and bring us children into their arguments. I had three brothers, but I was really lonely. I'm fighting for it not to be like that for my boys. They get the raw end of it. They're Mummy's boys and they can pick it up when I'm down. My eldest was a very withdrawn, difficult child. He never smiled. He never laughed. I feel so guilty about that. He was very unhappy and a lot of other people noticed that. He used to say, 'Stop it' when I was crying. Then he used to go out into the garden and shut the door.

I'm glad I've got them. I get love from my children. The little one was born with the cord around his neck and wouldn't breathe at first. I hated him at first. I would have loved to have had a girl. When I came out of the anaesthetic — he was born by Caesarian section — I couldn't believe it. I wouldn't give him any maternal love at first. Then somebody told me what had happened and how he struggled to breathe and I felt dreadful. I didn't love him as much as I should have. But I've grown fond of him as he's got a bit older. I'd desperately like another baby, but my husband refuses. He says he's not going through all that again. I've got to stop thinking about it.

I find it hard to mix and make friends. I went along to the mother and toddler group once, but I was feeling down and no one spoke to me, so I didn't go any more. The only person I can talk to is this young lad who lives down the road. I've known him for quite a long time. I met him by accident one day and started talking. He's always said that, any time I feel down, it's fine to go and talk to him. He used to give good advice and you need to talk to get it off your chest. Talking to him did help. But he's young and doesn't really understand. Really it's down to you to help yourself.

Joanna's story

I was in my late 20s, recently married, and working for a stockbroking firm in London — in fact, I'd been responsible for setting up the London branch of the company — when we decided to have a family and I got pregnant. I had a perfectly normal pregnancy and worked until two weeks before the baby was born, though I was absolutely huge. We'd recently moved from London to this lovely new house in the country. I had a straightforward delivery and everything seemed to be fine.

But then, there I was in this new house with a new baby. Or rather, I wasn't. Because I was never in the house. The minute he woke up in the morning I used to put him in the car and drive off somewhere, and only come back at night to put him to bed. The only time he slept during the day was in the car whizzing up and down the motorway. I was going up to London three times a week to see girlfriends. I had plenty of friends, so I made sure I was out all the time. I used to go out to restaurants for lunch and he would sleep in a sling.

Another stupid thing I did was when he was four weeks old: my husband had to go to Paris on business and I went with him, taking the baby. I must have been mad — everyone told me I was mad, including my husband. While he was out on business, I remember pacing round the streets of Paris with this tiny child in a sling, not knowing where to go to feed him or change him. And I remember being in this grand hotel, feeling trapped with this baby. I should have had help then, but I didn't think.

I didn't have a very good GP at the time. Every time I went to him during the pregnancy he did nothing but complain about the amount of weight I was putting on. I wasn't eating huge amounts or anything like that, but I just billowed out like a balloon. I put on four or five stones, but he did nothing constructive except moan about it.

The baby always looked immaculately dressed. People always used to say how marvellous he looked but his mother was a total wreck, hugely overweight. I was all alone and my husband was working very hard so he wasn't home much. I will always look back on Tom's babyhood and think that I didn't enjoy it. He was quite demanding, but I'm sure that was because I was always stressed and tense. I was always worried that something might be wrong with him. With my second child, well, he brought himself up. I mean you know that they're not going to die at the slightest thing. And he consequently is a totally different child — very laid back.

I had no experience of small babies. I went to all the classes and they all talked about the magic moment of giving birth, but not a word about the tiny child. It wasn't that I missed work, I'd no intention of going back, I hated it.

Whenever the baby woke up in the night, my husband just snored his way through it. He was absolutely useless. I've got girlfriends whose husbands go and make tea for them in the middle of the night and keep them company. The other thing was that I didn't let him cry. The minute he cried, I picked him up. Then once I was so fed up I just put him down and let him cry and left him for about half an hour and he was still crying. When I went in, the child was just covered from head to toe in sick . . . he was drowning in it. He was only a couple of months old then and I felt so dreadful that from then on he didn't cry again. We used to just pace up and down trying to get this wretched child to go to sleep. Poor baby, he probably needed to be put down and tucked in firmly. I mean, we probably kept him awake jiggling him up and down. I used to do that for two or three hours at a time.

Round about seven or eight months, he started waking up in the night, and then I did find it really difficult. But my health visitor was quite helpful and we managed to get him off that. No one at any time suggested there might be anything wrong with me. I think they all put it down to my being a new mother.

Then, suddenly, when Tom was nine months old, I went to a girls' luncheon. I was very quiet and somebody said to me — someone I didn't know very well — 'Are you alright?' and I burst into tears. This girl said: 'Do you think you're suffering from post-natal depression?' I sobbed my way to the doctor's and he said: 'Oh, yes. Your trouble is you're a workaholic!' and he gave me some pills.

My husband didn't realize there was anything wrong because he just wasn't around. He would come home late at night and then Tom would always start crying. He always cried while we ate and one of us would end up holding him. It didn't occur to us to stick him in his room until we'd finished. It was always tense and I used to feel resentful. I didn't think it was my fault. When he came home, my husband was tired and just wanted to relax.

I didn't know anyone else who suffered from post-natal depression. There was one girl I met in hospital who had her baby at the same time, who said she felt depressed, but she wasn't a close friend, so we didn't talk about it. All my friends either had older children or didn't have them at all and it was never mentioned. During the NCT (National Childbirth Trust) classes, no one ever mentioned PND at any point.

I took the pills my doctor gave me for a couple of months and began to feel better. Then I thought, 'this is ridiculous, I can't go on like this,' and I stopped taking them.

Tom was always a very clingy child and I took him absolutely everywhere with me. I remember we went abroad on holiday and it was absolutely ghastly from beginning to end. I remember going to the mother and toddler group and he used to just sit on me and he wouldn't do anything. I loathed going until I met this one girl I could be friends with but then I didn't go any more.

My health visitor used to come round every week — she was wonderful. She always thought that Tom was awkward and I was always phoning her up to ask her advice and she was great. But she seemed to think it was because I was a new mother with a new baby. Looking back, I was putting on a very good show. But no one ever asked how I was feeling. You're just expected to carry on. It's non-stop with babies. You can't even go to the loo without a child tagging along and if they're clingy like Tom, then they end up sitting on your knee while you're doing it. I just couldn't relax or anything.

I left it for ages before getting pregnant again. I think I was worried about being depressed again. I couldn't cope with two young children close together — I don't know how people do. It's hard work being with children, much harder than going out to work. I don't think men understand that. They have no idea what it's like. My husband still gets cross when he comes home. 'Why haven't you done this? Why haven't you done that?'

I thought in fact I might have got depressed after having Ben because right about the time I was due to deliver, my husband said he couldn't stand commuting any more, so we got a flat in London where he stays all week, coming home only at weekends. There I was, alone with two children, but fortunately I got a nanny and I did find it easier. It was nice just to have the freedom. I love the children dearly and I've now met a nice crowd of girls with children of a similar age and it's great.

My sister reckons our mother had post-natal depression. I think probably what saved my mother was that she had to go back to work. I remember when I brought Tom home, both my husband's parents and mine were appalled by this demand feeding. They used to say to me, 'God, you're not feeding that baby again!' I breastfed him for seven months without any problems.

With my second baby I was hugely overweight again and I was selfish this time, I didn't breastfeed him after the first few weeks. He's two now, and I still don't think I've fully recovered, but I'm getting better.

The strange thing was that of course I'd heard of post-natal depression and read about it in magazines, but I just didn't think it applied to me. It was only at that luncheon when someone mentioned it that it suddenly seemed obvious. I knew I wasn't happy, but I'd got this wonderful new home, this lovely baby and everyone kept saying: 'Aren't you lucky?'

When post-natal depression is a serious illness

The most severe form of post-natal illness, puerperal psychosis, is quite different from the other forms of the condition. The next case history illustrates how a victim's behaviour becomes so altered that there is no question of coping with life and hiding the illness from the people around her. Nor can it be passed off as something that all mothers go through. It is quite clearly a severe mental illness, but fortunately the outlook for those who suffer from it is excellent. Hospitalization is almost always necessary but, once treatment is begun, recovery is assured.

Marilyn's story

It happened after the birth of my second child, which seems strange really because, if anything was going to happen, you would have thought it would have been with my first which was unplanned and which, really, I wasn't very happy about. But with my second I'd waited five-and-a-half years until we felt the time was right and she was a much-wanted and properly planned baby.

The first birth was perfectly straightforward with no problems. The second, though, was very quick and all so sudden that I didn't have time to have any pain relief. The first was bearable, but the second was so much worse although it actually took only two hours. It was a short, sharp shock. And although it was a girl, which we wanted as we already had a boy, I remember I didn't feel as elated as I should have. I thought I would be more thrilled about it.

She was a wonderful baby, no trouble at all. In fact both babies were. There were no problems. I fed my little boy myself for 10 months, but I only managed to feed Amy for 2 months because I was so ill. What started it all was her name. It wasn't popular with the family. I began to worry about how to spell it. Should it be the English way, or the French way, or some other way. Finally I narrowed it down to a choice of two spellings but I just couldn't think about anything else.

This problem about the name had gone on for a long time. When we told the family what we were going to call the baby if it was a girl, they were horrified. My mother actually drew up a list of names which she liked: 'Why don't you call her Catherine?' she said. And she told me that my sister had actually said that she wouldn't call the baby by the name we had chosen. In fact it was a long time before she used the name. And she never picked up the baby and cuddled her for a long time. My family are very snobby and they didn't think it was a middle-class enough name.

Back at home from hospital, I was aware that things weren't right. I suddenly felt very depressed. I couldn't cope. I didn't have any enthusiasm for anything and I think I had this fixation about the name so that I wouldn't have to think about the baby. I was literally changing my mind every two minutes. At that point I thought that if I could get the christening over with, and the name problem sorted out once and for all, then it would all be all right.

I was so worried about this name that I couldn't sleep and then my milk supply dried up. So then I began to think, 'oh dear, I can't be a proper mother if I can't feed my baby' and that replaced the name as my fixation. It snowballed and became a major disaster in my mind. At that point my mother said that I needed help. She may have been a pain to start with, but she was absolutely marvellous when I was ill. Both sets of parents were very good — they needed to be.

I went to my doctor and he gave me some tablets to take, but I hated the idea of taking drugs. My head knew it was right, but my heart wouldn't let me, so I didn't take the full course. I remember we were going out one evening and I wanted to have a drink and I knew that I couldn't drink with these tablets, so I flushed them down the toilet. It was the worst thing I could have done.

I started to go backwards then. I got worse and worse, more and more depressed. I used to love being on my own, or going shopping, things like that and I couldn't do them any more. I couldn't bear to be alone. I used to haunt other people's homes. I used to go from house to house. I was full of self-pity all the time, it must have been awful for the people I visited.

Everything was black and white, there were no shades of grey. The amazing thing was that I could see what was happening to me, but I couldn't do anything about it. I was such a pain. I got a variety of responses from people. A nurse told me to pull myself together, but there were others who listened to me. But I used to compare myself with everyone else and they were coping wonderfully. I wanted to be them. I hated me. I used to think, if only I could be Paula or Sheila or whoever it was. They're much better than me.

I was very hard to live with. Normally I'm quite good at cooking, but I couldn't even work out what to do for a meal. I tried to work out menus for six months at a time for some reason, and I couldn't do it. I hated shopping. I resented having to cook and shop. I would burst into tears just listening to some song on the radio.

This went on for about six months. Then I started having psysical symptoms. I got a pain in my stomach and it got so bad that in the end I had to stay in bed and have someone here with me. I wasn't eating and if I did I used to go upstairs to be sick. I was almost anorexic. I was violently ill if I travelled in the car. There were about two hours in the afternoon when I didn't feel ill, so I used to look forward to that. Afterwards it would all come back.

I tried to kill myself twice. The first time I was at my mother's house. I went out into the garden and just thought, well, I'm doing everything wrong, what's the point? I nibbled some rowan berries from a tree and there was a rush of adrenalin as I thought, 'I'm going to die'. The ambulance rushed me to hospital and then they found out what I'd taken and it turned out they weren't poisonous.

Another doctor came to the house to see me and, though I was depressed that day, he didn't seem to take me that seriously. I said I didn't want to take the drugs and he made a joke about it. But I was really ill. My GP wouldn't admit that he wasn't coping with me and he said to my mother that I wasn't that ill. But I was putting on an act for him. My mother tried to tell him this and say that I wasn't normally as well as this.

The second attempt at suicide was more serious. I'd managed to cook a meal for my parents the night before. I'd done quite well and was feeling pleased with myself. Then I had this adrenalin feeling and I got a handful of pills and put them all in my mouth. Fortunately they were sugar-coated and they made me feel ill, so I took them out and went round to a neighbour and told her I'd done this very stupid thing, so she rang the ambulance. All this time my little boy was downstairs playing with a friend.

Another neighbour came with me in the ambulance and I must say there's nothing like being close to death to make you realize how much you want to live. It was a cry for help really. I wasn't getting any help then and things were getting worse and not better.

They insisted that I should go into a psychiatric hospital and I realized then how much I loved the baby. I couldn't have her with me, though, and that didn't help. A lot of the people there were really very strange and I remember trying to help one young man. In a way it helped me. I was there for a week, but it wasn't very nice. I saw various doctors and I must say I wasn't very co-operative, but they weren't very sympathetic. I kept asking if I would ever be cured and they wouldn't tell me. In the end I discharged myself and they were obviously quite glad to see the back of me because I was such a nuisance. One doctor accused me of being insincere.

I came back home and I shouldn't have done because I wasn't cured and I couldn't cope. Our mothers used to take it in turns to look after me. I was aggressive and hostile and though I never took it out on the children I began to think: 'Supposing I might do something to them? Supposing I'm not really safe?'

I used to talk and talk the whole time. I used to wander round the house after my mother talking the whole time about whatever my obsession was. In the end she used to scream at me because there was just no way to stop me. I used to threaten to go down to the railway line and throw myself under a train. I did it all the time. Sometimes I used to walk out of the door and slam it behind me and someone would have to come after me. Sometimes I used to wake my husband up in the middle of the night, just talking about whatever my latest obsession was. Some days I used to phone him every five minutes at work. I would put on foreign accents, hoping they wouldn't realize it was me. Fortunately they were marvellous about it all. I let myself go totally and I remember almost deliberately making myself look awful. I used to have the most horrible sadistic thoughts about killing the baby, and get sexually excited by it. It sounds dreadful, but I couldn't help it. I didn't dare tell my doctor about that because I knew he wouldn't understand.

In the end I was desperate to find somebody who could treat me. I tried a hypnotist, all sorts of things, but nothing worked. Then I pleaded with my father to find the best doctor in the country to cure me. And he found a psychiatrist for me to see privately. I gave her my version of things although I was almost too ill to talk to her and she got in touch with my father to say that I must go into hospital. It was in the nick of time. I think I was slowly dying.

I was taken into a private hospital and it was like somebody waving a magic wand, for the psychiatrist told me that what I had was treatable, that I would get better. She told me she guaranteed it. I was given hope and it makes all the difference. The trouble is with most doctors that they won't commit themselves, they're so anxious not to say the wrong thing. But the fear of the illness is much more frightening.

I was in that hospital for six weeks, heavily sedated at first. The baby was with me though a private nurse looked after her at the beginning because I just slept most of the time. Then I was given ECT (electroconvulsive therapy) and it was wonderful, I felt so much better. It was like a big black cloud being lifted from my head. I had 12 or 13 treatments in the end. I used to look forward to them because I felt so much better afterwards.

When I eventually went home, I was still on a lot of drugs and the doctor warned me that the tranquillizers I'd been taking would have side effects. For instance, our sex life was stone dead. And then the drugs were addictive, so I had withdrawal symptoms, but I was prepared for those. They said to me, if you can recover from the depression, then you can manage the rest. It was a bit like taking two steps forward and one back. I did have a couple of relapses when I had to go back and have ECT, but I was almost becoming addicted to them. They made me feel so good that I had to stop.

Now we're virtually home and dry, but it's taken two years. I do feel that I missed out on time with the baby. But I see it as the least important time of all. She wasn't aware of what was going on, although I didn't want to pick her up and cuddle her. I couldn't enjoy her. My son knew exactly what was happening because there were occasions when I was really horrible and spiteful to him. But my husband explained that it was because Mummy was ill, that I didn't really mean it. And he seemed to understand. I heard him say the other day, 'When Mummy had post-natal depression . . .'.

Looking back, I was very anxious as a child. At 10, I got so worried about an exam that I suddenly couldn't walk. It was psychosomatic. Then when I went on to convent school I hated it there because there was very sophisticated bullying. Both me and my sister had to see the child psychologist when we were children. I remember when I was in the psychiatric hospital I wanted to see what was in my notes, so I managed to sneak a look and it said there that I had pushy parents. I suppose they were. Both my husband's mother and my mother are very dominating. He had a breakdown of his own some time before mine, so he was always very understanding and supportive, even through the worst parts because he knew what I was going through. Now we've learned to stand up to our families more and not to let them interfere and to do what we want to do rather than what they want us to do.

I just feel now that the doctors let us down. My father had to spend thousands on private treatment and I should have been in hospital a lot sooner than I was. I wish there'd been a mother and baby unit I could have gone to in the beginning. I feel my GP couldn't cope but didn't dare say so. Another thing is that such a rosy picture is painted of what childbirth is going to be like and it's so unrealistic. I went to NCT classes and post-natal depression was never mentioned. They build up this image of how the birth is going to be, and in my case it was unbearable. You end up feeling inadequate. And I wish I'd been able to talk to someone else who'd suffered from it. I felt worse because I thought there was only me and everyone else was coping.

Obviously Marilyn's case was very severe. She was suffering from the most serious and fortunately quite rare form of post-natal depression, post-partum psychosis. I have included her experience to illustrate a case of full-blown mental illness as well as the illustration of what most sufferers experience.

CHAPTER TWO
Defining depression

For the vast majority of women suffering from post-natal depression, if it is recognized at all, it is often underplayed and dismissed as just one of those things all new mothers go through. This attitude seems particularly strange when you consider that the condition has been recognized in legal terms for many years. In British law, under the Infanticide Act of 1939, for example, a mother cannot be found guilty of the murder of her own child within 12 months of childbirth because 'the balance of her mind is disturbed by reason of her not having fully recovered from the effects of giving birth.' A mother can, however, be prosecuted for the less serious offence of manslaughter of her child, though this is extremely rare.

Perhaps one of the reasons why PND has so long been neglected by the medical profession is that it falls between two specialties, psychiatry and obstetrics. Neither feels particularly at home with it and the vast majority of both psychiatrists and obstetricians know little about it. So what seems to happen when a mother behaves a little strangely on the post-natal ward is that it is often assumed that sending her home will solve the problem. There she comes under the charge of her family doctor, and he or she is the one left with the responsibility of deciding whether her condition merits treatment.

There is yet another factor to consider here. It is widely accepted that PND affects about one in ten new mothers. But research shows that only a very small percentage of these women are diagnosed as suffering from PND, let alone receive treatment. It is equally obvious therefore that the majority get well on their own. Perhaps even more importantly, as the case studies given here show time and again, the majority of post-natally depressed women do not even realize they are ill. They put their feelings down to the change of lifestyle they undergo with a new baby and the extra work involved. And the nature of the 'illness' is such that they blame themselves and their own inadequacies for not coping when they see everyone around them glorying in motherhood. Worse still, the condition is often mistaken by those around the victim for laziness, or a bid for attention, selfishness or downright ingratitude, to which the common response is 'pull yourself together' from both relations and, sadly, professionals alike.

There is a wide array of symptoms related to PND, but one specialist in the field has said that often the easiest way to detect a depressed person is to ask: 'How are you feeling?' and when the response is to burst into tears, a very common reaction, then quite clearly there is something wrong.

The following are some of the common symptoms, although by no means all victims will suffer from all of them: bouts of crying, feelings of panic and an inability to cope, feelings of inadequacy, extreme tiredness which even a good night's sleep fails to alleviate, an inability to concentrate or think clearly, forgetfulness, general aches and pains, and a feeling of being unwell for which there is no other cause, unnatural gaiety, indifference to the baby, insomnia, feelings of utter despair, thoughts of suicide, loss of appetite or craving for certain foods, loss of interest in sex, being unaware of the baby's needs, complete loss of energy.

If you have recognized yourself or someone you know in what you have read so far, then there are two very important things to remember. First of all, you are not alone, others have felt and are feeling just the same as you. There could well be another mother you know feeling just like you, but like you, hiding it very well from the outside world. Secondly, you are suffering from an illness for which you are not responsible. You have not done anything to cause it and it has absolutely nothing to do with your ability as a mother. It most certainly does not mean you are a bad mother. Thirdly, you will get better. It may take some time, but one morning in the not-too-distant future, you will wake up and realize that you can see light at the end of the long dark tunnel, or that the black cloud is lifting and you will realize that you are beginning to feel a bit better.

The different post-natal illnesses explained

The conditions that make up post-natal illness are grouped into four main categories: from the mildest 'blues' to the most severe puerperal psychoses with PND itself and the other, less common, post-natal disorders fitting somewhere in between.

The 'Blues'

The term post-natal 'blues' is restricted to the passing weepiness, depression and irritability that the majority of mothers suffer in the first two weeks after the birth of a baby. Although the blues clear up of their own accord, the condition can sometimes herald the start of a more prolonged post-natal depressive illness. It has been known throughout history and has been given various names: the maternity blues, the three-day blues or the five-day blues, and was once commonly known as milk fever because it was thought to be associated with milk coming into the breasts.

The most common symptom of the blues is crying and this is accepted by health professionals dealing with the new mother as a part of the whole process of giving birth. But it can be very distressing, even embarrassing, for the mother who 'knows' perfectly well that she should be feeling happy and contented with her lot.

Around 80 per cent of all new mothers experience some symptoms to some degree: as well as crying these can include feelings of irritation and anger as well as feelings of hostility towards the partner or even the doctors and nurses looking after the mother.

Most doctors agree that the basic cause is a change in hormone levels. Throughout pregnancy hormone levels rise to accommodate the growing baby and by the time labour begins, levels of progesterone and oestrogen are 50 times higher than they were before the pregnancy.

After birth these levels fall suddenly and dramatically so that within hours, the levels of progesterone and oestrogen can have dropped to below what they were before the pregnancy began. Dr Katharina Dalton, also known for her work on premenstrual syndrome, has done much work on the subject of PND and hormone levels and this is dealt with in more detail later in the book in Chapter 3.

The blues, although usually a passing phase, should not be dismissed in quite the way it is, because it can give an indication of more serious depressive illness to come. Professor John Cox in his book *Postnatal Depression, a guide for health professionals*, writes:

> 'Particular attention should . . . be given to those mothers with severe blues who are known to be at increased risk of postnatal depression because of a history of psychiatric disorder, or a strong family history of mental illness. Such mothers should not be discharged home in an aroused emotional state, but kept in hospital to ensure that their mood has not deteriorated. If they insist on going home it is important that primary care workers are informed that they are likely to become depressed so that additional domiciliary care and early treatment can be initiated if a serious psychiatric disorder develops.'

He goes on:

> 'It is beneficial if the midwife listens carefully to what the mother is worried about, and allows her to express irritation with the family, the baby or with the staff. It is unhelpful to dismiss such a mother's distress as "just the blues", because this trivializes a painful emotional disturbance; to respond to such a mother by being irritated or "arguing back" is also not therapeutic.'

Other post-natal disorders

Although it is generally accepted that depression is the most common post-natal illness, other conditions which can also cause much distress include phobias, hysteria, anxiety neuroses and obsessive or compulsive neuroses.

Agoraphobia, where the mother fears crowded places, is not uncommon and when a mother is too frightened to leave her own home or to go into crowded shops, serious problems can arise. How, for example, can she visit the baby clinic or even her own doctor? Fortunately agoraphobia can be treated by a variety of behaviour therapies once the mother has been referred to a suitable specialist such as a clinical psychologist.

One of the most common neurotic disorders is anxiety neurosis. This condition carries with it a number of unpleasant symptoms such as headaches, sweating palms, palpitations, restlessness and sleep problems. The mother often worries so much she finds it difficult to get to sleep or she may have panic attacks or suffer from hyperventilation, a form of rapid breathing that can make anxiety worse. Again the key to solving such problems is sensitive treatment including psychotherapy and learning to relax.

Obsessive and compulsive neuroses are not quite as common but they are just as distressing because sufferers are so caught up with repetitive rituals such as checking windows or doors, or hand-washing, that the routines of looking after a baby are severely disrupted. The mother may also have aggressive thoughts and these can be very distressing. Again, however, behaviour therapies can be very helpful and the outlook for recovery is very good.

The puerperal psychoses

As we saw earlier, in Marilyn's story, puerperal psychosis is a very severe illness, but it is also uncommon. It is thought to occur in at most two or three cases in 1000. One of the most frightening things about this condition for the mother (as illustrated in Marilyn's case) is that she often realizes that her behaviour is abnormal although she is powerless to do anything about it.

● Many sufferers have delusions either about themselves, the baby, or the people around them. They may be very restless, constantly walking about or talking and they often have pronounced mood swings; insomnia is also a common symptom. Some mothers have even been known to try and kill their own babies because they may believe that the child is evil in some way; others may try to kill themselves.

● Fortunately, because such obviously abnormal behaviour cannot be hidden, it is impossible for this psychotic condition to go undetected. Treatment may necessitate a stay in a psychiatric unit, and the mother is seldom able to care for her baby without considerable help and support. There are a number of mother and baby units for the treatment of this illness and some mothers find this form of treatment particularly helpful and preferable to separation from their baby.

One British doctor, Dr Margaret Oates in Nottingham, has developed a different approach to treating post-natal depression. She has set up a community service so that mothers can be helped in their own homes and this has been working for some time with considerable success. While it is obviously cheaper to provide such a service it is also, for many mothers and their families, a much simpler and more convenient way of dealing with this particular problem.

Post-natal depression

The major problem with post-natal depression is that although a mother is the focus of attention from health professionals for quite a considerable length of time after the birth of her baby, the condition is still very seldom recognized and diagnosed.

Mothers who are feeling depressed are often very reluctant to tell anyone how they are feeling. They feel guilty because they are not happy. They may have strange thoughts about wanting to harm their babies or themselves and worry that if they confide in anyone, they may risk losing their baby at worst, or being thought of as a bad mother at the very least.

Some depressed mothers visit their doctors regularly with a variety of symptoms that they do not themselves realize are linked to depression. They may have problems sleeping or eating, or some other difficulties. They may have tried to confide in someone and been told to 'pull themselves together'. This is still a very common reaction.

A depressed mother is very often giving out signals all the time about her condition. She is often excessively anxious about the baby and how she is coping with it. She worries about feeding, whether she has enough milk or whether bottle feeding would be better for the baby. She worries about the baby being ill and she is often over-protective and overresponsive to the baby. Many depressed mothers avoid going to the baby clinic or to other social groups because they feel inadequate alongside a group of other apparently happy, contented, coping mothers and because they fear that they may be criticized for their handling of the baby. Depressed mothers will always have a good reason for not being able to do something, but the reason will seldom be a positive one.

The most common symptoms are a feeling of being depressed. This sounds obvious, but very few mothers will themselves report this. It is only when they are questioned directly: 'Are you feeling sad and depressed?' that they will admit to it. A disturbance in the sleep pattern is one of the most common features of the illness. It is understandable how this can often be overlooked as an important symptom when the new mother's sleep pattern is bound to be altered by the very fact of having to adjust to the baby's feeding requirements. But it is not normal to have difficulty getting off to sleep, or to wake up early in the morning for no obvious reason.

Depressed mothers feel inadequate, incompetent and guilty and no amount of reassurance can convince them that they are coping well with the baby. Some mothers worry that the mother-baby bond is not present, that they do not love their babies enough or even at all and a mother may say that she has no feelings towards the child. Some mothers start to have thoughts about harming themselves or the baby and are very reluctant to confide these thoughts for obvious reasons.

Depression is also a common cause of loss of interest in sex although there are many other causes for this after having a baby. If other factors such as infection after an episiotomy (where a cut is made in the perineum to facilitate birth) or simple fatigue have been ruled out as the cause, then it could well be depression.

Tiredness is probably the most common symptom of PND and depressed mothers will describe it as a feeling of complete exhaustion. Some mothers of babies who are either ill or have sleep difficulties and whose own sleep is thus seriously disturbed will also feel exhausted, but it is relatively simple to differentiate between the two. The depressed mother will find that rest has little or no effect on her. No matter how much rest she has she always wants more. An exhausted mother will, however, feel much better after a few undisturbed nights.

Mothers on the other hand who feel depressed and have two or more of these symptoms present for longer than two or three weeks should be considered as possible sufferers from post-natal depression.

CHAPTER THREE
What we know about post-natal depression

Post-natal illness was first written about by Hippocrates in the Fourth Century BC, and it is amazing to think that post-natal depression was one of the first psychiatric disorders to be recognized. The most serious form of the illness has been recognized for almost 200 years. It was often described in early psychiatric literature and yet its causes are still not understood. All this has prompted one expert in the field, Dr Channi Kumar from the Institute of Psychiatry in London, to question why it is that when between 500 and 1000 women are being admitted to mental hospitals every year within the first few months of giving birth, people are not jumping up and down and demanding to know what is being done about it. Dr Kumar goes further. He has said that if men were known to suffer from the condition, there would be a lot more done in the way of research to discover the cause.

There is now no doubt that this can be a very serious illness and as we have already seen, few women are forewarned about it. Although many women obviously become very ill, their numerous and often severe symptoms appear to go unnoticed. This is at a time when they are at the centre of a network of health care: they are seeing doctors, nurses, midwives and health visitors. No wonder, then, that partners and relatives of victims find it hard to be sympathetic and accept that there really is a problem.

The sad thing is that although doctors have made childbirth itself a very much safer event than it used to be for both mother and baby, there has been little or no impact on the incidence of post-natal depression.

This situation is slowly beginning to change. In recent years there has been a considerable amount of research worldwide into the subject although it is probably fair to say that Britain leads the world as far as current knowledge about post-natal depression is concerned. In the early 1980s, a group of British and other interested psychiatrists founded the Marcé Society, named after the French psychiatrist Louis Marcé who first wrote about post-natal illness in the mid 1850s. For many years his was the only comprehensive study of the illness in the world. The aim of the Marcé Society is to promote research and knowledge of the illness. At one of their early conferences it was agreed that the first step was to stop puerperal psychosis being classified along with other psychoses and to give it an identity of its own.

Separating PND from other depressive illnesses

Most books, magazines, publications and classes for pregnant women, if they bother to mention the subject at all, dismiss PND, usually mentioning only 'the blues' in terms of something most women suffer, which goes away very quickly, and which is nothing to worry about. No wonder then, as many of the women interviewed in this book illustrate, that a depressive illness was not something they considered to be the cause of their symptoms.

Research, too, has not always been helpful. One study carried out a few years ago compared the incidence and type of psychiatric illness found in women during the post-natal year and at other times. The doctors concluded that there did not seem to be any difference between the two groups. This begs the question does post-natal depression exist? Another doctor went on to show, using exactly the same statistics, that the illness very definitely does exist, pointing out that the incidence of psychiatric disorder was staggeringly high during the first three months after the birth of a baby.

Perhaps one of the most interesting findings in recent years has been that the illness is not confined to Western cultures. Research done among African communities has shown a striking similarity in incidence, calling into question the confident assertion in one pregnancy and childbirth handbook, and echoed in many others, that 'in a supportive environment geared to helping new parents before, during and after a birth, post-natal depression is virtually unknown; in modern society, however, depression is more common.' It goes on: 'The incidence of emotional difficulties after birth can be greatly reduced when the natural process unfolds without disturbance.'

Some years ago the cause of post-natal depression was also linked to concern about the increasing use of technology and medical intervention in the process of childbirth. It has also been linked to arguments about whether birth should take place at home or in hospital, the changing role of women, and the loss of family support. In the early 1970s, two doctors in particular, Arms and Shaw, put forward the view that before the development of modern obstetric practice, childbearing had not been associated with suffering and pain. Others have suggested that post-natal depression is in fact found only in Western culture because of these modern developments.

But Professor John Cox found in his research in Uganda that African women did in fact show signs of post-natal depression and that many of the symptoms suffered by their counterparts in the West were similar to those described by African women. Ten per cent of the women in the studies had a post-natal depressive illness that usually began within two weeks of the birth; symptoms were distressing and disabling and usually lasted for several months. Home and hospital deliveries were compared but childbirth in hospital was no more likely to be followed by depression than a home birth.

What causes PND?

Researchers divide into two main camps on this issue. On the one side are those who are looking at psychological and social factors which might be implicated in the condition, and on the other there are those working to find a biochemical cause, that is, something which happens within the body's own mechanisms to cause the illness. There are generally speaking three main arguments. Firstly that PND has nothing to do with childbirth but is something which happens to a woman who is vulnerable psychologically. Secondly, that the psychological stress involved in becoming a mother is the cause. Thirdly, that it is due to physical changes in the body caused by pregnancy and childbirth.

The study that confirmed beyond doubt that there was an increased risk of psychiatric illness following childbirth was carried out in Edinburgh by R.E. Kendell and colleagues in 1981. By surveying thousands of women they made the important discovery that there was a 16-fold increase in the likelihood of a mother being admitted to a mental hospital three months after giving birth compared with any of the three month periods from one year before the birth to one year afterwards. Depressive illness was by far the most common mental illness suffered.

Professor Brice Pitt in London then investigated further and came up with the estimate that around one in ten mothers were affected by post-natal illness. This figure has been confirmed many times since by other studies, and experts see it as a minimum estimate.

The role of hormones

The body's activities are controlled by hormones, the chemical messengers whose job it is to make particular cells in the body act in a certain way. Hormones control, for example, growth, digestion, excretion, temperature, and all other bodily activities. Most importantly as far as PND is concerned, they also control the female functions of menstruation, pregnancy and birth. The principal reproductive hormones are oestrogen and progesterone, as well as prolactin which is responsible for the production of milk.

The pituitary gland, situated at the base of the brain, and linked to the hypothalamus, the brain's nerve centre, is responsible for initiating the production of these hormones. Within hours of conception, the presence of a fertilized egg is beginning to affect the levels of hormones. Oestrogen and progesterone levels rise throughout pregnancy — up to 30 to 50 times higher than at any other time — and there are specific hormones which appear during pregnancy which are not produced at any other time. The menstrual 'clock' which has previously controlled these hormones, becomes dormant, and the placenta and the fetus take over control.

At birth these hormone levels, which have taken months to build up, abruptly drop and within hours they have become a fraction of what they were. Then there is a period of rest before the menstrual cycle starts up once again and re-establishes control of the reproductive hormones.

Dr Katharina Dalton, in her book *Depression After Childbirth*, feels that there is a link between PMS and post-natal depression. She comments:

> '*A mother's normal adjustment to such marked changes in hormonal levels is indeed heroic, and one wonders at the large number of women who can stand up to the changes without upset, rather than express surprise at the few who are disturbed by this hormonal upheaval.*'

Dr Dalton has had some success in treating depressed women with progesterone, but this is not the end of the story. Unfortunately we do not yet know exactly what the normal levels of hormones are in women, although research into this continues. But Dr Dalton comments:

> '*The proverb says "the proof of the pudding is in the eating" and progesterone has been successfully used in the treatment of post-natal depression.*'

This treatment is undoubtedly still controversial, but, in its defence, Dr Dalton points out:

> '*The idea that hormones can cause psychological disturbances is not new, there are many examples in medicine. The adult with too low a hormonal output from the thyroid gland may be referring to the psychiatrist because of depression, apathy, slowness of thought, inability to concentrate and confusion. The mind is sick, but the cause is hormonal. Similarly, the individual with too high a thyroid level may go to the psychiatrist with agitation, nervousness and restlessness and be incorrectly diagnosed as having "anxiety neurosis", but the illness may be corrected by lowering the thyroid level.*'

Dr Dalton goes on:

> '*The evidence which suggests that post-natal depression is*

of hormonal origin relies firstly on an understanding of the tremendous hormonal changes which occur during pregnancy and the puerperium and the ease with which these various hormonal levels could be put out of balance together with an awareness of the limitation of our hormonal knowledge . . .'.

Some mothers find that the hormonal changes in pregnancy can be so marked as to trigger mental disturbances, although for the majority of PND sufferers, it is the birth itself which is the crucial factor.

Dr Dalton is not the only one to have looked at hormonal levels. One team of researchers from the University of Oxford studied hormonal blood levels in a group of women in late pregnancy through until after the birth. The team also used a questionnaire designed to detect depression. Beyond any doubt, they found that those women with the greatest drop in progesterone levels after delivery were those most likely to say they felt depressed within 10 days of giving birth. This research also uncovered the fact that the group of women who felt depressed after the birth also included more women who suffered from PMS.

Why then are hormone levels not measured routinely? Unfortunately, the answer is that it is not very easy. Doctors still have much to learn about normal hormone levels and what affects them in ordinary day-to-day living so the procedure for such testing is at present complex and expensive. Hopefully, in the next few years, these problems will be sorted out.

The next case history, Elaine's story, is interesting because she was herself convinced that there was a physical explanation for her experience of depression. She is also one of those relatively rare women who begin to suffer during pregnancy and go on to suffer after the baby is born.

Elaine's story

I had three girls, 6, 4½ and 20 months and we really wanted to have one last try at having a boy. I really enjoyed being pregnant with the girls, I'd loved it all the way through. We tried for a while and nothing happened so my husband decided to go for a vasectomy. He had to wait six months for that, so we kept trying while he was waiting and finally I got pregnant. Right from the beginning the whole pregnancy was just awful. It didn't feel the same at all. At about seven months I had a terrible bout of flu and really felt ill. I went on feeling like that for a long time. Then one morning I woke up — the children were on half-term so all three were at home — and I just couldn't settle or sit down I felt so restless. I realized later that it was a panic attack. I phoned my husband at work to come home I felt so bad.

From then on it got worse and worse. I was anxious, I couldn't sleep properly and in the end at 34 weeks I went into premature labour and had to go into hospital. They thought it was a medical problem. I was worrying about how small this baby was going to be but the labour stopped and they did all sorts of tests to try and find out what it was but in the end they said it was just one of those things. I had a dreadful panic attack at the hospital because I thought they weren't going to let me go home. I was just sitting on the edge of my bed looking over my shoulder and feeling awful.

Nic, my husband, took a couple of weeks off work and somehow we muddled through. We couldn't understand why I felt so ill and anxious. I felt like throwing myself out of the window. I just didn't care. I remember sitting and trying to work out which window would be the best to jump from. I used to say to myself: 'Now pull yourself together.' One moment I felt well, really good, elated in fact, and the next I was really down. The fluctuations worried me.

Then, once I was home, I suddenly went crackers in the kitchen one day, screaming, shouting and shaking all over. Nic phoned round everyone, the hospital, the GP, midwives, and one of them said it sounded like post-natal depression. The doctor came round and offered me tranquillizers, he said they'd keep me calm until the baby was born. Once I'd had the baby, he said, I'd be all right. But I thought, no thanks I don't want any pills, I've seen what happens with that sort of thing.

I was a nurse and towards the end of the pregnancy I started thinking about hormones. I used to get hot flushes and a friend said that her mum was getting them because she was going through the menopause, that's what made me think. When it was mentioned to the doctor, he just laughed. The GP did mention it to the consultant, but he couldn't see how the hormones could get mixed up like that during pregnancy. In the end they put it down to my being a neurotic mother.

All my three other children had to be induced, so when I got to term with this one I begged them to induce me straight away. I wanted to get it over and done with so that I could get better. The labour was a bit strange and everyone commented on how quiet I was. I couldn't feel the contractions until I actually wanted to push. The pain wasn't registering, it was like a mental block because I was so far down with the depression. I remember seeing that he was a boy and shouting that out to Nic.

When I went down to the ward, I was just at rock bottom. I remember looking at him and thinking it was a boy, so it must have been worth it. But the normal elation wasn't there. I was over the moon with my other babies, even when with the third, we'd wanted a boy, I was still absolutely thrilled to bits. I'd always wanted to hold the others all the time, but I didn't with him. The doctor who'd induced him realized it was depression, but he said it would only last for four to six weeks after he was born and then it would get better. But it didn't.

I wanted to get out of hospital as soon as I could and they sent me to see the social worker. They told me to take the baby with me and I knew they wanted to see how I was with him. But in the end the social worker turned out to be a good ally. His wife had just had a baby and he understood how women felt. It was good for Nic, too, because he had another man to talk to who understood. Once we got home, instead of getting better, I just got more and more depressed. I was panicky, anxious, claustrophobic. I used to go for long walks. They started to talk about post-natal depression, but when I went to see one of the doctors in our practice, he just said, well I've known you through three other pregnancies and there's no reason why this one should be any different. He told me much later that he just didn't know what to do. He'd never seen PND so bad before. He did come back several times to talk to me and he put me on vitamin B6.

Then at the six-week post-natal check, he put me on the contraceptive pill and it had an immediate effect. I felt terrible. I knew straight away what it was and I made an appointment to see him. When I went along to the surgery I just stood in the waiting area, banging my head against the wall. The receptionists just looked at me. They thought I was a nutter and they didn't know what to do. When I got in to see the doctor, he took one look and said I should go home, have a nice cup of tea to get myself together and the psychiatrist would come and see me. I staggered out of there and looked around for somewhere to go. Straight across the road was the convent where I'd gone to school so I went there. It was a sanctuary. I was screaming and throwing myself about but there was a nun there who had trained as a counsellor. She was used to dealing with drug addicts, anorexics and people like that and though she'd never come across anyone like me before, she just sat and talked to me. She was so kind, and I left there feeling much better.

Once the psychiatrist came, I was so desperate I would have done anything. I was quite happy to go with him to the hospital, but my dad got really angry and refused. He said there was no way I was going to the mental hospital. He told Nic he was going to take me and the baby home for my mum to look after — because that was the other thing, they wouldn't let me take the baby to hospital. So they gave me anti-depressants and let me go home.

My mum was very good. She'd always had a tendency to take over, but she didn't this time. She stood by me and watched what I did and made sure I looked after the baby properly. It was very frightening for her because she'd never experienced anything like that before and I'm sure she was worried how she'd cope. I wasn't sleeping properly. I slept more in the day than at night, but I was only taking half the anti-depressants I was supposed to. The children used to come and see me every couple of days and it helped just to have the baby to look after.

The baby was on the bottle by now, because though I thought he'd been feeding well, one day I realized that he hadn't had a wet nappy and when the nurse came to see him, she realized I just didn't have any milk at all. I'm sure that was hormonal, too.

After a few weeks I was able to go back home again. The two older ones were at school, so I used to walk down to my mum's with the little ones and stay there all day. My father would pick the children up from school and then Nic would come and collect us after work and take us all home. It must have been very hard on everyone.

There was a friend close by who was very good and who would come and sit with me sometimes when I was on my own. I filled my week with as many things as possible, getting out and seeing people, so I wasn't at home alone. I used to go and visit relatives and people I wouldn't normally dream of visiting just to get out. It was a question of taking a day at a time.

My confidence had completely gone. I felt I was no good to my family, that the children didn't need me, that I was totally useless. I quite often used to run off intending to jump off a bridge. Once I was running up and down the middle of the dual carriageway in a complete panic. I used to head for the nearest woods and hide sometimes. In the house I used to imagine throwing the baby on the floor and it swallowing him up, or I used to see hands coming out of the walls and taking him away from me. I would cry and rock backwards and forwards. Most of the time, outwardly, I used to carry on as if everything was normal but once I cried on my youngest daughter's shoulder and she wasn't even two at the time. She just laughed and hugged me better and said 'Mummy, don't cry'. I felt dreadfully guilty about it.

Nic had to have lots of time off work. Fortunately he wasn't very far away and he would always come home if I asked which I did a lot. Sometimes he'd come home for just an hour and then go back. He must have got into trouble about it, but he never said anything. Sometimes I used to get in such a state that I'd scream and shout and send the children to bed without any tea. When Nic came home from work, he'd have to sort it all out.

In the end I got so desperate, and I'd been on and on about it being hormones, that I phoned Katharina Dalton's office. I spoke to her secretary who was very kind and managed to fit me in very quickly. She insisted on seeing us both together and she spent most of the time explaining to Nic what was happening to me and why. He came out of there feeling so relieved. Beforehand I'd been going on month after month about it being hormonal and I'm sure it had crossed his mind that I was becoming obsessed about it and I think he began to wonder, is she really going mad?

I started progesterone treatment and within a week the anxiety and panic attacks were easing off. Once I'd started my periods again, it had settled into one long dreadful cycle, but after one month, I realized that I felt better. I still felt quite bad but the symptoms were relieved and I felt more able to cope. Slowly, slowly I began to get better. Now after 16 months, I'm cutting down the progesterone gradually, so that in six months' time I'll be off it completely. It's a long process. I never used to worry about my periods, I was always regular and never had any problems, but now I get very bad PMS.

I suppose it has affected my relationship with my son in the sense that he's a Daddy's boy. Before I went to my mum's Nic was looking after him most of the time. He was the one who got up in the night to give him his bottle. I think it's nice now that they're so close. I don't notice that I feel any differently to him than I do to the others. It was just something that happened and I don't blame him for it.

Looking back at the pregnancy as a whole, the signs were all there, lots of little things, but nobody saw them. I get very angry sometimes when I think about it. It was so obvious. Now I bombard my GP with information about PND, and I know he's treating some of his patients suffering from PND with progesterone to see if it helps. We've got a small group going and we meet for tea with new mums and their babies. There are quite a few with PND and a couple of quite bad cases.

My advice is to find somebody, anybody you can talk to sensibly if you have this. You don't want someone fussing around. It doesn't matter what other treatment you have, you need to talk and get it out of your system. The nun I used to see regularly was wonderful. She made me see that the treatment wasn't going to do it all for me, but that I could get through. I was very lucky. Every time I had a session, I used to come out of there feeling good about myself. She used to tell me how well I was coping, how strong I was.

My eldest daughter used to cry sometimes that she didn't want Mummy to die. But I don't think now that the children remember much about it. We protected them as much as we could. But it's hard to hold back and keep yourself under control when you feel like that. It's hard trying to cope when you just don't want to.

Are some women more at risk from PND than others?

For some years it was thought that the length of labour or complications during the birth could be implicated in PND, but recent studies which have looked at these points, fail to find any such link. It was also thought that single mothers and mothers from lower social classes were more at risk. Again, this is not now thought to be the case.

Other lines of research have looked at the idea that certain social or psychological factors may be involved in PND. There have been several studies demonstrating that this can be the case. One study highlighted anxiety during pregnancy, marital dissatisfaction, the lack of a close confiding relationship and previous PND, all of which could be risk factors.

Work has been done which demonstrated that a woman who has had difficulties in her relationship with her own mother, may find it difficult to believe in herself as an adequate mother. It has also been shown that women who were deprived of attention in their own childhood had a greater difficulty settling into the role of mother. Interestingly, women whose mothers were not around at the time of the birth of their own child, either because of death or family separation, were more likely to suffer post-natal illness than those whose mothers were able to visit or make contact in some other way.

Another recent theory on the cause of depression is that a woman who has always had a view of herself as incompetent and therefore often suffers from depressive feelings, will not be able to cope adequately with childcare, and will as a result develop a secondary depression. However, often women who have been successful and confident in their career find themselves shocked that their skills don't transfer to coping with the baby and they, too, can suffer from post-natal depression.

One of the most interesting recent research projects has been to develop a simple questionnaire to be given to women as part of their ante-natal care which will predict those women who are most likely to suffer from PND. This work is being funded by Birthright, the mother and baby charity, and is being carried out by a clinical research team in Cambridge. They are aiming for a diagnostic technique and treatment which will be of practical use to those health professionals working closely with women in the post-natal period.

The psychologists are concerned that quite apart from the considerable distress the illness causes to the woman and her family, research has already shown that the condition can in some cases damage the relationship between mother and baby and also have an effect on the development of the child.

Dr Lynne Murray, one of the members of the research team, first became interested in PND when she was doing a straightforward developmental psychology study in Edinburgh. Quite by chance she noticed that one of her volunteer mothers who had become depressed behaved in a completely different way to the other mothers. She went on to study 700 depressed mothers and their children and found that a clear picture emerged of the mental state of the depressed women.

Dr Peter Cooper, a lecturer in psychopathology at Cambridge, has been involved in a study of nearly 500 mothers. Both doctors found that almost none of the women suffering from depression in their groups was spotted by the health professionals dealing with them. They are currently setting up another research programme with 4000 mothers to try out a new ante-natal questionnaire which they are developing for use in the last three months of pregnancy. This will hopefully be used to detect those mothers who are at risk of suffering from post-natal depression. Says Dr Cooper:

'There are a lot of non-specific factors which give rise to depression at any time, things like a poor marital relationship, poverty, lack of a confiding relationship, and stress. If any of these are present at a time in your life when you have more demands on you such as the general demands to do with caring for an infant: less sleep, in addition to all the rest, it's not surprising you become depressed. Specific problems may arise in a group of people who themselves have had unhappy childhood experiences where their own dependency and needs have not been met, and who are then faced with caring for a being who is totally dependent on them. It may be that this provokes a depressive reaction. We have to look into this in much more detail to discover what the vulnerabilities are.'

The second stage of this exciting research is to then develop a treatment which can be integrated into post-natal care. There is already a wide range of treatments available, but the researchers' idea is to treat the difficulties arising between mother and child as a result of the depression. The hope is that they will be able to offer psychotherapeutic treatment within the NHS. The project started in 1989 and is expected to take three years; it is also hoped that their results will lead to a new approach to the problem within the community in about five years' time.

Research is also going on to try and develop a biological test which would confirm PND, but this is a long way off. In the view of Dr Peter Cooper, though, there is no problem detecting depression. The problem is that while a woman who has recently given birth is subjected to the attentions of a whole battery of medical experts, examining, prodding and probing every physical aspect of childbirth and its aftermath, seldom does it occur to anyone to ask after a woman's emotional well-being. Dr Cooper feels that two or three sensitively asked questions could remedy that situation. And, hopefully, in the not-too-distant future that is exactly what will happen.

CHAPTER FOUR
The importance of the birth experience

Women approach childbirth in a variety of different ways, but there are very few who sail through pregnancy and childbirth without any misgivings about the process and how they will cope with it. The most important question in a woman's mind is 'What exactly is it like?' Unfortunately there are hundreds of variations on the answer to this one, and very seldom are women given the right one. For the only honest answer is that other women can only tell you how it was for them, no one can tell you how it will be for you. And that applies whether it is your first or your tenth baby.

Women want to know: 'How will I know when labour begins?' 'How much will it hurt?' 'Will I be able to stand the pain?' 'What can I have to ease the pain?' 'When should I call the midwife or go to the hospital?' 'How long will it last? . . .' While there are obviously particular signs and symptoms to look out for, and certain stages that everyone has to go through, it is impossible to answer the other more personal questions because everyone is different and every birth is different. A lot of unnecessary worry, which can lead to serious problems later, is caused by people who, undoubtedly with the best of intentions, give women unrealistic ideas about childbirth.

The emotional minefield

There are two extremes. At the one end are the doom and gloom merchants, those women who are all too keen to describe horrific stories of pain and terrible anguish, laced with plenty of gory detail. At the other are the fanatics, clutching their birth-plans as if they were the Ten Commandments, making strident demands about how they would like their birth to be, what they will and will not have, and how they will not deviate one jot from this ideal. They forget in their fervour that the point of all this is to be safely delivered of a healthy baby.

In between are the vast majority of women who have read a little, talked a little, worried somewhat, have been to relaxation classes (usually only for the first baby because it has not proved so easy in subsequent pregnancies with a toddler in tow), and who by the end of nine months are anxious to get the birth over with, so that they can get on with the important part of it all — bringing up their child.

This is not to underplay the importance of the experience, and certainly not to underestimate the emotional minefield in which a woman finds herself during the first few days and weeks after the birth. Rather, it is to underline the point that the birth is only the beginning of a long journey into a relationship with a precious new person. It is certainly not the climax of the experience, which is how it is often described. It was very striking how many of the women interviewed for this book complained that although a great deal of time and effort had been spent preparing them for the birth, very little if anything had been said about the period immediately afterwards. As a result, they felt let down, betrayed almost.

This is a common fault in the huge array of books available on the subject. They take you in great detail through every little nuance of pregnancy and childbirth and then stop. And most of us who have bought these books suddenly find that when it comes to the everyday worries and problems we encounter with a new baby, the bible we have clung to for months is no longer any use. We are in the dark and on our own. So we then rush out and buy a baby book. But there is usually a gap there, too. Most of these devote little space to those all-important days and first weeks after the birth when you need to know whether it is normal for a baby to sleep for hours on end, or whether it is normal for a baby not to sleep for hours on end, and a host of other questions.

I well remember bringing my own first child home from hospital on a lovely warm summer's day. Following the hospital's strict instructions to make sure he was warm enough, I firmly closed the window in his room, switched on the heater, dressed him in several layers of warm clothes including a hat and mittens and swaddled him in several blankets. I did have some doubts about this procedure, especially as it meant stripping off most of my own clothes before I could bear to suffer the temperature in the room. But I was following the hospital's instructions to the letter — after all, they knew best. Fortunately I did have the sense to check with my health visitor, who went to look at the room. She was horrified and immediately switched off the heater, flung open the window and took most of the bedding off my poor, sweating baby. This was quite a common fault, she told me, adding that she could not understand why hospital staff seemed to be under the impression that everyone in the world outside lived in sub-zero temperatures.

It was an easy mistake to make, for like many new mothers, I had had little or no experience of brand new babies. This is a common situation these days and one example of how motherhood has changed in the second half of this century.

Preparing for the birth

Conception is no longer the haphazard event it once was. Although it cannot be denied that there are many unplanned pregnancies, for most couples these days, having a baby is usually a carefully planned and conscious decision. Once it has happened, then it's off to the doctor and into the system. There follows the routine of hospital and clinic visits, regular checks and tests, and the decision about which sort of classes you want to attend in preparation for the birth. While some women are quite happy to leave all the decisions about the type of birth they will have to the doctors and midwives — and it must be stressed there is nothing at all wrong with that approach — others want to take those decisions into their own hands.

Whatever you have decided to do, during the last weeks of pregnancy some, though not all women, feel relaxed and confident and look forward to the birth on the one hand although at the same time, they may feel apprehensive at the approach of the actual birth experience. As you contemplate the impending birth you will quite naturally have many thoughts about the kind of experience ahead; some of these are listed below:

Hopes and fears

You may worry as the date draws nearer that you may not be able to live up to what you would like to think of as your own or anyone else's expectations. The best way of dealing with this fear is to try and approach things with an open mind. You will have prepared as well as you can, through reading and classes, you are fit and well — hopefully — since you have attended all your regular check-ups, and what you must do now is to keep an open mind. Many women, ideally, would like a pain-free, natural, quick birth, and for the vast majority, although it may not be quite so straightforward, it is at least different from how they feared it might be. Whatever happens during your birth, producing a healthy baby is a wonderful achievement in itself.

How will my body cope?

As you grow larger and larger towards the end of pregnancy, it seems almost impossible to believe that the baby will be able to make its way through the pelvis and vagina and out into the world. Sometimes these fears are compounded by the fact that you may have had a previous difficult birth or simply because it is your first pregnancy. Nature usually takes care of these problems, but the best way to deal with them is to read about the processes of birth and if you have any worries, talk to your doctor or midwife who will be able to reassure you. You will also find that relaxation exercises will help you feel more confident.

Handling the pain

This is a major concern to most women. The way to deal with it is to ask the professionals who will be helping you with your birth what methods of pain relief are available and to discuss them. If you are one of those women who feel strongly that you want a completely natural birth and have made preparations for this, don't make the mistake of closing the door completely on pain relief. Keep your options open, it is no less of an experience and you are no less of a mother because you changed your mind and had to be helped to cope with the pain.

Losing control

No one knows how they will react to the birth experience and, as well as worrying that your waters are going to break in the middle of a supermarket, women worry about losing control and shouting or making a lot of noise and about the whole experience of baring your most private self in front of strangers. Most hospitals, midwives and doctors are perfectly understanding about this, but this is where a partner can be particularly supportive. Make sure your partner knows your feelings and is prepared to make them clear when you may not be in a position to do so. And though it may seem like a contradiction, losing control is exactly what you have to do during labour, allowing your body to take over.

Medical intervention

After hearing horror stories, many women worry about the use of forceps, or having an episiotomy, or simply about the use of monitors during the labour. The best thing to do is to ask about the policy of the hospital where you will give birth, and if you feel strongly about a particular issue, then ensure that your views are recorded on your notes. Most hospitals these days are happy to handle the birth in the way the mother wants it as long as everything is going well and there are no complications, and as long as she has talked about it calmly with the staff first. Problems usually only arise when women make strident demands and lay down the law about what they will and will not have. If you have discussed your views sensibly with the staff and you have found them unhelpful and obstructive then perhaps you should consider an alternative birth place. But all these problems should be ironed out beforehand. It will help neither you nor your baby if there is a clash of ideas in the middle of the labour.

The birth itself

It is undoubtedly one of the great medical success stories of this century that infant mortality rates and the mortality rates of women in childbirth have been cut dramatically. But at the same time there was a period in the late 1970s and early 1980s when medical intervention was becoming routine and was often unnecessary. Generally speaking, that situation has begun to stabilize and we are moving back to a far more balanced approach to birth.

A number of studies have been carried out to see if there is a link between post-natal depression and the birth experience. But none so far has succeeded in showing this. It is probably the case, however, that while an unpleasant experience may not actually cause PND, it does not help the mother's state of mind and can lead to unhappy feelings of guilt and inadequacy.

Induced labour

This is a very common experience for women, although again it is not quite as common as it was just a couple of years ago. Apart from any other considerations, it is often very difficult to know exactly when the due date is and the mother's own dates and those of the hospital frequently differ. Many women are not aware that they can resist induction if they feel strongly about it, and many hospitals are quite happy to let a pregnant woman go past 'the due date' if she tells them she would rather wait for labour to start naturally and there are no medical reasons why this should not be the case: i.e. mother and baby are both well. Some consultants will only allow a woman to go past that due date by a few days, others will give it three to four weeks.

Acceleration of labour

This can either be done by rupturing the membranes or by the administration of a drug. It can be useful if you have been labouring for several hours to little effect, or if the baby is becoming distressed, but interference in this way can speed up the contractions to a much more intense and painful level.

Episiotomy

This is a procedure where the doctor or midwife makes a cut in the perineum in order to make the outlet for the baby larger. Again in certain cases it can be a great help, but recent research shows that when comparing episiotomies with situations where the perineum is allowed to tear naturally, the latter heal much more quickly and effectively. Both, however, lead to the need for stitches and this is why episiotomy has often been labelled 'the unkindest cut of all'. Problems following episiotomies are more common than many doctors either like to admit or even realize. If you are still feeling sore by the time you have your post-natal check at six weeks, then you should seek help, either from your own doctor, or by asking to be referred to a specialist.

Forceps delivery

Here special birth forceps are used to speed delivery in cases where the baby is showing signs of distress. The idea is to help the baby out as quickly as possible if for any reason you are unable to push it out yourself. Professionals often put a time limit on the second stage of labour, after which you are thought to be in need of help. It is worth asking your attendants whether by a huge effort to push you will be able to help yourself and manage without forceps, and sometimes adopting a different position, such as kneeling or squatting, can give you the extra push you need. The latest research also shows that when comparing this method of assisting with the lesser-known vacuum extraction, the latter is less punishing for both mother and baby. But different hospitals differ in their practice and again it is worth checking beforehand if this is something you feel strongly about.

Caesarian section

This is sometimes an operation which saves either the mother's or the baby's life, and while it is fair to say that no doctor would perform a Caesarian section without some indication that intervention might be necessary, the numbers of sections done has been steadily increasing and has led to some questioning of the use of this procedure. In America, particularly, there is no doubt that many obstetricians view a Caesarian section as a safe, acceptable alternative to what they see as a potentially difficult, possibly dangerous, and sometimes impossible vaginal delivery. Some women may find it a relief to be able to avoid the pain of labour, but others feel cheated out of what they see as a rewarding experience. So, if one is offered to you, you must check why your doctor feels it has to be done.

Is there such a thing as a 'good' or 'bad' birth?

It is still quite fashionable to talk in glowing terms about 'pain-free' natural childbirth. According to its exponents it is simply a question of learning how to control your body through relaxation and other exercises. But for some women, no amount of preparation has spared them from an excruciatingly painful labour which left them demanding anything and everything the doctors could give them. On the other hand there are those women who did not bother with any advance preparation at all and who sailed through the whole thing in a very short time with no pain relief at all.

As Virginia Ironside says in her book, *How to Have a Baby and Stay Sane*:

> 'The truth is that some births are agony and some are marvellous, and some are a bit of both, and "relaxing" has barely anything to do with it. (Obviously those who did classes and had marvellous births claim that there is a relation between them.) Some ante-natal classes can quite spoil the birth with their unfulfilled promises of ease and "naturalness" and make mothers who don't experience pleasure feel guilty into the bargain.'

One of the biggest complaints which women make is that neither the midwives nor the doctors would listen to what they had to say about what was happening to them; this is particularly so with first-time mothers. The problem has undoubtedly been that as birth has become a more hospital-based practice, midwives have lost their status and much of their unique input into birth has also started to be lost. Unfortunately, too, along with this has gone a decline in the number of home births. Hopefully now, though, the tide is turning and it is gradually becoming easier for women who do want the experience of home birth to have one. For, to many consultants' consternation, research shows that, far from home births being more of a risk to mother and baby, in many instances they are actually safer than in hospital.

Michel Odent, the French obstetrician, questions the interference of many consultants in the process of childbirth and believes that hormones play a key role here. He argues that given the right set of circumstances — a peaceful, calm, relaxed setting — a woman's hormones will take over in the vast majority of cases to produce an effective, natural childbirth. He feels strongly that midwives have a key role to play and questions many of our present-day practices, particularly where men are concerned.

Childbirth is a very personal experience. Some women want to labour naturally and welcome the pain they suffer as a part of this process. Some women fear and dread the process and the pain and want anything that modern medicine has to offer to alleviate it. When considering the long-term effects of all this on the mother herself, the important thing is whether she was allowed to make her own choices and whether her wishes were respected wherever possible. If they were not, then there should be valid and fully explained reasons why this could not be. The important thing is that conditions are such that women are encouraged to make their views and feelings known, whatever they might be, in the knowledge that they will be respected and listened to.

CHAPTER FIVE
When partners become fathers

Everyone must have heard by now about 'new man'. He's a truly wonderful creature: loving, caring, considerate and kind right from the beginning of a relationship, but he comes into his own when his woman becomes pregnant. He is just as thrilled as she is about the whole thing, from buying baby clothes, to decorating the nursery, to waiting for hours with her at the ante-natal clinic. Of course, he joins her at all the classes, is fascinated by every detail of the experience she is undergoing, and of course is thrilled at the prospect of being with his partner at the birth. There is naturally no problem about taking time off work for the big day, no question about not being there to support her every twinge. With the arrival of the baby, he has no problems with changing nappies, helping out at home, cooking meals, ironing shirts and chipping in with the housework, and of course, gets up with his partner during the night to make cups of tea.

There are, no doubt, one or two of these amazing creatures about. But the vast majority of women have to make do with a man who is probably quite pleased about the prospect of becoming a father, but would really like to escape the technical details. He may come to the odd preparation class under protest, feeling rather uncomfortable, and he will be with you at the birth because that is the way things are these days. After the celebrations are over, it comes as a bit of a shock to most men that life then doesn't return to pre-baby normality.

But this does not mean that men don't want to become involved. The fact is that despite all the talk of equality, shared care, paternity leave, etc., it isn't always easy for men to devote as much time to their partners and children as they would like. Like it or not, we still live in a society where men are seen as the main breadwinners. The majority of women who return to work after they have had children, do so because they need to, to help out with the family budget.

In their book *Kitchen Sink, or Swim?* written by Deidre Sanders with Jane Reed in the early eighties, the authors wrote:

'*What happens to a child in his first five years very much affects what he is like, what contribution he will make to society and his chances of happiness, for the rest of his life.*

In general, children would be happier, more balanced, more healthily independent, fulfil their potential better and be less likely to become delinquent if they received more of their father's time and attention . . .. If fathers were generally involved in the care of their children from when they were tiny, this would encourage warmer, closer bonds between father and child. Some men might find it an effort to get involved in the very physical, tactile world of a small baby, but so do women faced with their first baby . . ..

With both parents spending half their "working time" doing their paid job and half looking after their child or children, the quality of care the children would get from each parent would be improved. They wouldn't consistently see dad and mum either only at the end of eight or more hours at work or else irritable from the lack of contrast and outside stimulation that being house-bound can induce.'

Little has changed in the years since those words were written. Except perhaps that most people accept that it would be better for everyone if fathers played a bigger role at home. But in practical terms, it just isn't possible for most people. It usually happens that at the point at which they become fathers, men are also at a crucial stage of their careers. This means that they have to balance their role as breadwinner with their role as parent. Fatherhood itself paradoxically also ties men more closely to their role of breadwinner. They now have dependents and gone is the option to throw it all up to sail round the world. It is now much more difficult for a man to give up a good, well-paid job just because he doesn't enjoy it. For many men who don't appreciate it at the time, it is a great sadness when they later realize how much they have missed as their children have been growing up.

Sharing the birth

It is now commonly accepted that men will attend the births of their children. In fact it has now almost become obligatory and this in itself can cause problems. For some it is not a happy, fulfilling experience which enables them to forge a wonderful, close relationship with their child from the very beginning.

Some men, quite understandably, find it difficult to cope with a situation in which their partner is suffering greatly and they are unable to do anything other than hold her hand. Some find the physical side of childbirth, the blood, the needles, the knives, the whole experience, very unpleasant and upsetting. There are some men, on the other hand, who become so involved with their partner's labouring that they almost take over, following the textbooks to the letter and insisting that she struggle through with no pain relief, just by breathing properly.

Michel Odent was one of the first specialists in the field to notice that some women were actually inhibited by the presence of their partner during labour, and managed much better when he was not present. In his book *Primal Health* Odent questions this new practice.

'*To dare ask such a question is almost scandalous at a time when childbirth is thought of as something just between a couple. But, having observed thousands of couples, who come from every kind of socio-economic group, it seems that things are not so simple as people think. The kind of bond between couples and the kind of intimacy they share can be incredibly different. The anxiety which fathers feel about birth is very different from one man to another . . .. The behaviour of some men during childbirth is perhaps more akin to the behaviour of primitive man. Men like this often play a positive role. They keep themselves in the background, sometimes even outside the room, as if to protect the privacy of their childbearing wives from the world outside. Perhaps behaviour like this is not very different from how it used to be in the primitive societies of hunter-gatherers: the men kept guard, protecting their women from the outside world and protecting the birth of their babies.'*

He takes his argument further and asks why it is that for thousands of years childbirth was always seen as something which women did in private with only other women present.

'In traditional societies, women shared their daily lives, and shared intimate things with each other, such as when they were having a period. So when a woman gave birth, the presence of other women with whom she was already intimate was not felt as a disturbance. In contrast some Western women can only find privacy in the bathroom . . .. There are some things which a labouring woman does which she would not usually do in front of her sexual partner. For example, during childbirth a woman needs to empty her rectum.'

Odent goes on:

'Another reason why it might be necessary to keep the worlds of men and women separate is to maintain sexual attraction. Sexual attraction needs an element of mystery . . .. Nowadays, in our unisex society where there is little distinction between men and women, the element of mystery has almost gone. I have been taken aback by the large number of divorces and separations among couples who shared marvellous birth experiences. On the other hand, couples where the man was not an active participant in the birth of his children seem to still have solid relationships.'

While many people would not perhaps go so far as Odent, he makes an interesting point. For it is true that in the same way as women are now pressured into trying to achieve a drug-free, totally 'natural' birth, men are pressured into being actively involved in a process which many find disturbing. I remember witnessing the spectacle of a group of women (some of whom had never themselves experienced childbirth) attacking a male friend who had announced that though he would support his wife through the early stages of labour, he did not want to be present at the birth itself. He was accused of deserting his partner in her hour of need, being a coward, and so on.

Sharing the first weeks

Once the baby is actually born, there is another area of contention. What part should a man play in the day-to-day care of his offspring? If a child is being bottlefed, there is absolutely no reason why a man cannot do everything for the child that a woman can. But in most family groups, women tend to take the lion's share of this task. In most instances, of course, this is the only way it can be because the man is out at work all day.

Some men still regard babycare as women's work and take little or no interest in a new baby. In the same way that some women find it difficult to get enthusiastic about a small, smelly, noisy bundle, it is the same for men. The majority of men are even less likely than women to have had any contact at all with tiny babies and often find the whole business of handling them very intimidating. Obviously if they are interested and want to handle their babies, then they can be helped and encouraged to do so.

There are cases, too, where women feel that motherhood and all it entails is their role and some unconsciously discourage the father from being involved, preferring to take the full burden themselves. Some feel that the man's role is to work to provide the wherewithall to keep the children. And men can feel very awkward in a situation where there is a group of competent and able women. Many new fathers feel positively neglected by — even jealous of — partners who are suddenly completely absorbed in the baby, although many either cannot or will not recognize this.

For women who feel that their partners are not taking an active enough role in caring for the baby, it is best to do something about the situation before resentment builds up. To begin with give him time to adjust to the new situation. He probably thought about the practical consequences of starting a family a lot less than you did. Talk to him about the baby, the new routine, the tasks involved. Work out how he can help, but don't be unreasonable. If he has to get up early either to face a stressful day in some high-powered city job, or a gruelling day driving a lorry up the motorway, then is it fair to expect him to get up in the night, too? Perhaps he could take over the night turns at weekends, so that you can get some sleep. It is important that at least one of you gets enough sleep — though not necessarily the same one all the time.

And don't be afraid to change the baby's routine around once you get home from hospital. Just because baby's bath time was fixed at 11 am in the hospital ward doesn't mean it has to stay that way. Make sure that your partner gets some of the more rewarding experiences with baby, too. Save bath time until last thing at night. Do it in front of the fire when everyone is warm and comfortable and hopefully relaxed so that you all enjoy it. And who knows, it may well mean that it has a soothing effect on the baby and make him settle and sleep more easily.

Is there sex after childbirth?

While there is no doubt that some marriages can be very happy without a good sex life, there is no arguing with the fact that a satisfying sex life can enhance a relationship. At a time when this special closeness would seem most appropriate, with the relationship cemented by the birth of a child, for many couples it becomes a bone of contention.

Most women lose all desire for sex for at least four to six weeks after childbirth, and some for a lot longer. Her partner, on the other hand, is looking forward to the resumption of sexual activity and finds it hard to understand her lack of interest. There are a number of reasons why many couples find it difficult to resume their normal sex life and these are outlined below.

The delivery itself

Even if you had a straightforward delivery, did not need an episiotomy and had no tearing, both of which need stitches, you are still likely to feel sore for about 10 days or so afterwards. Feeling so bruised and battered, you cannot even bear to think about sex until your body has healed. This may take a little time, but be assured you will feel comfortable again. If your first attempt at intercourse is uncomfortable, it may put you off even more, so it may be as well to make sure you are completely healed before attempting it. Women often find that lubrication is a problem for some months after the birth of a child. But this can be easily remedied by using a suitable proprietary lubricant. If dryness is a problem for you, don't suffer in silence because it will only make the problem worse. If you have any worries about this, mention it to your health visitor or your doctor who will be able to advise you. It is not unknown for an episiotomy repair to be done too tightly and so cause problems later. If intercourse is still painful some time after delivery, and you feel this could be the reason, you should talk to your health visitor or doctor about it and get help.

Fear of pain

Many women are simply afraid that after the experience of childbirth, sex is bound to hurt. If you feel this way, talk to your partner about it and take it very slowly and gently until you feel comfortable. You may also have decided that you don't want any more children, and this may subconsciously affect your attitude towards sex. Again talk to your partner about this and make sure that you are using some form of contraception, even if you are breastfeeding. This can offer some natural protection against conception after giving birth, but it is by no means guaranteed, and there are many breastfeeding women who have become pregnant within a very few weeks of delivery.

Feeling tired

This is something that every mother feels. It is quite normal, there is little you can do to escape it completely, and it is no reflection on your ability to cope. It is quite unreasonable of a man to expect you to be his enthusiastic lover when you have been on the go all day and up several times during the night coping with the demands of a hungry baby. But it is hopeless expecting him to realize all this on his own. You must sit down with him and tell him how and why you feel as you do and exactly what this new 24-hour-a-day job means. He should then be happy to help out with the chores, with the baby, and make sure you have some rest. If you have a partner whose attitude is that babies are women's work and sex is your duty to him, then it is going to take a little more concentrated effort. You are going to have to make him aware of just how demanding a tiny baby is. Perhaps he would agree to take charge of the baby for a day while you go shopping. Or he might be encouraged to take over the night shift one night at the weekend. Most men appear insensitive to these problems because they really have no understanding of them. For your own sake, it is important that you try and make him understand.

Fighting the flab

It can come as a great shock when you wake up the first morning after your baby's birth to discover that there is still a huge mountain of flesh wobbling about all over your stomach. Most women imagine that this somehow disappears miraculously, and for the lucky few this is the case, but the majority of women have to work at it. The next shock comes when you find you cannot get into your pre-pregnancy jeans to leave hospital. Then, after the initial euphoria, you begin to feel down: your skin looks terrible and your hair falls out. In other words the bloom of pregnancy seems to have disappeared overnight. On top of that you get home and are surrounded by the smell of nappies, sick, and milk, and there seems little point in putting on nice clothes just for the baby to ruin. Feeling good about yourself and sexual desire usually go together. To improve the situation, you need to devote some time to yourself. Get someone to look after the baby while you go and have your hair done. Buy something nice which is not baggy but which actually fits. Find a babysitter and go out with your partner for a candlelit dinner, or even arrange for your mother or someone close to keep the baby overnight. Your baby will not suffer. You are not neglecting him and it most certainly does not mean you are a bad mother.

Babies, babies, nothing but babies

In the first few weeks after the birth, it is quite natural to be wrapped up in this new responsibility. And there is no doubt that it will affect your social life. Not everyone will be delighted if you turn up at their party with a carry cot. But don't become totally overwhelmed and refuse to do anything unless the baby is included. It can be a difficult adjustment to make for a couple who have previously both enjoyed interesting jobs and an active social life to find that one partner has no conversation except feeds, nappies and gurgles, to the exclusion of all else.

Is it any wonder men resort to clearing off to the pub night after night? Of course men can be unreasonable and expect you to be the same carefree woman as before, able to throw an impromptu dinner party for six and take it in her stride, or who could get herself looking wonderful inside 10 minutes to join him for a drink at the pub. But don't always automatically say 'no' to everything he suggests, or he will soon stop asking.

Post-natal depression in men

There is some evidence to suggest that perhaps fathers, too, can suffer a form of post-natal depression. Of course, they do not suffer the serious illness that some women go through, but the change in their lifestyle and role can lead to stress and depression and this is seldom recognized for what it is. Little work has been done on the impact of the birth of a child on a marriage, and it does not feature at all on the list of stressful life events which can lead to crises. But the Tavistock Institute in London has done some long-term research into the effect of a baby in the family and has come up with some interesting findings.

One great problem is the current fashion for the caring, sharing, do-everything-together partnership which can be very unsettling for those couples who do not fit the mould. The birth of a baby, no matter how much wanted and planned, changes the relationship. A woman suddenly has this small creature who demands her full attention and to whom she transfers all her mothering. Her partner is often left feeling resentful and jealous towards the baby who has taken over his position in his wife's affections. She senses this and can even begin to feel contemptuous of his feelings and attitude. Add to all this the fact that while her lifestyle has changed substantially, his own remains largely the same with, most importantly, no curbs on his freedom, and it is easy to see how the partnership can founder.

At a time when we are beginning to look seriously at the changes that a woman has to undergo in her life, perhaps it is time too to consider the problems that men face in taking on their new role as parent. This is vital, not only for them, but for the women who are their partners.

CHAPTER SIX
Housebound and helpless?

Is there any way to avoid post-natal depression? This is a pretty tall order, and a presumptuous one, but there are certainly ways that you can make things easier for yourself during the early weeks and months after the birth. You may have spent hours decorating the nursery your new baby will occupy, getting his or her clothes ready, attending the ante-natal classes, and reading everything you can lay your hands on about childbirth. For some strange reason very few women actually give much thought to the practicalities of coping with a tiny baby. Because of the way our society is organized, the majority of women have had little more practice with a baby than a quick cuddle with a friend's or relative's child. In other words we are quite inexperienced in handling a new baby, let alone physically taking care of its needs.

This applies to the basics like changing nappies and clothes, to bathing, washing and cutting fingernails, never mind feeding. You were probably given demonstrations in the hospital on some of these points, but it is quite a different matter when you are left alone with no experienced nurse to help you out if you get into difficulties. And you may well find that to add to your problems there is an eagle-eyed mother-in-law watching you closely and with plenty of comments on how it was in her day. No wonder most of us rush off to the peace and quiet of a bedroom, where at least we can fumble away in privacy.

It really is quite unrealistic to expect any new mother to be automatically able to cope with her first baby. Even if you've been brought up with babies, or worked with them, it is quite different having one of your own to care for. There is a lot of talk about 'maternal instinct'. But even if there is such a thing it certainly does not include an inborn ability to do up babygros the right way.

In many cases, the birth of a baby can be perceived as a surprisingly disruptive event in a woman's otherwise well ordered life. A successful career woman, for example — as in the case of Carmen, below — may find that although she copes superbly with her job, when it comes to her new baby, things are not quite so easy for her.

Carmen's story

I was 29 and happily married when I had my daughter Daisy who's now two. I was working in television producing drama and my lifestyle was incredibly volatile, erratic and insecure. I travelled about a lot, quite a lot of it abroad. I had this naive view of what it would be like to have a baby, a romantic image of the baby fitting into my lifestyle. I was so sure that I'd be able to cope and would take it all in my stride that I had a trip booked for six weeks after the baby was due. I was terribly pig-headed looking back. I thought: 'I am strong, I'm a new woman, I can do it.'

I worked until three weeks before she was born and everyone thought it was amazing. In fact, some people didn't even realize I was pregnant, and I almost enjoyed that. I suppose I was almost denying the pregnancy in some ways. I was at a quite important point in my career and it was a fast lane sort of life.

The whole thing really came as a great shock. I went to NCT classes and listened to all this stuff about natural birth and thought it would all be lovely, but reality was quite different. My waters broke and then nothing else happened. I refused to go into hospital and spent three days at home holding out before I would go in. I went into the natural childbirth room, but still nothing was happening at all. They were trying to persuade me to let them help things along, but I kept refusing. Then they finally said that the possibility of infection was very great and that if that happened I might not come through it! We'd been waiting 60 hours by then.

It was very cruel, I felt, the way they ripped me away from

the quiet calm of the natural birth room to the technical room. I was no longer secure, I felt totally out of control, and I felt like the baby was being ripped away from me. There was a very horrid midwife who said, 'Oh, you're an NCT person, why don't you get on with it, girl?' I had an induction with a drip. It was supposed to be introduced at a regular pace, but she kept pushing the rate up and up. It was like torture, the whole experience was pretty awful. But when she was born I felt very powerfully in love with her from the first moment and I was completely euphoric for the first couple of weeks.

Then at home my mother had come to look after me and my husband was around too, and there was this big competitive thing between them. But everything was going OK until after about three months. I'd even managed to go on the trip I'd booked, then I'd taken on a lecturing job, which was full-time but meant that I had two hours travelling each way every day to work and back. Then, when she was six months old, we decided to move away because my husband got a new job and two weeks after we moved I became a totally different, desperate person.

It must have been happening gradually, but I hadn't really noticed it. Every morning I'd wake up and feel like all my nerve endings were exposed, like I was sitting on the edge of the world, but the rest of the world didn't know about it. No one else knew what I was feeling. When I walked down the street, I would look at everyone else and think that though it looked like a pavement we were walking on, I knew that if you jumped off the edge, it would be off the edge of the world.

I used to wander about the house, crying and crying. I would let Daisy stay in a dirty nappy for longer than she should and I felt dreadful pain at not being able to look after her properly. Then I'd sit in a corner and cower. When the cleaning lady came, I was so desperate, I made her sit with me instead of cleaning. I was still working, but I couldn't do the journey on my own and my husband was driving me to work every day in his car. I would sit there in the car and scream and say I couldn't face it, and he used to have to persuade me to go in and do it. I couldn't cope with anything to do with organization or order. I behaved in a most peculiar way and once ended up in my boss's office in floods of tears. I had to be taken to the doctor's. I didn't even know what I had in my handbag. I would stand in front of a group of students and think I don't know what to say to them. There were long silences and I wanted to die.

I had a searing sense of what I had done — bringing this child into the world. It was just horrific. I went to the doctor and he was just terrible. They sent me to a psychiatric hospital where I was put on anti-depressants. I saw a woman doctor and she said, 'Look dear, I've had four children and I'm a doctor, and we all know it's hard work, dear.'

It was just awful. I couldn't be in the house on my own. I had panic attacks. My next door neighbour was just wonderful. I used to be shaking and crying and I couldn't cope with looking after the baby, so she would take Daisy while I had a bath and changed my clothes. Then one day I was absolutely desperate. I felt completely mad and went round to her. She called the doctor out she was so worried, but when she came round and saw me, he was furious. He said that he could only be called out for emergencies and this wasn't one and he walked out. I ended up running down the street after his car crying and shouting 'please come back, please help me.' I was totally hysterical and he just drove away.

I phoned the Samaritans lots of times. I used to phone lots of people up. My husband's parents were wonderful and supportive and they used to come when I felt I couldn't hang on any more and they took care of the baby and the house. I went back to my old doctor who sent me to a psychiatric hospital and when I got there I went into a day centre and saw all the people there and the psychiatric nurses and I thought I'm nearly in here now. I couldn't talk to them and kept saying things just to get myself out of the door. Then I was in such a state I got on the wrong bus and when I got off I got an attack of the shakes in the middle of the street. I was paranoid about having something on my work record saying that I was unstable or mentally unfit.

In the end I contacted the Guild of Psychotherapists, the Women's Therapy Centre, and MIND and through them I found a therapist round the corner from where I lived. I had to go privately, and I was seeing him three times a week at first, but it gradually came down to once a week and that was the stabilizing factor. Even now I don't think I'm 100 per cent better, but I'm coping.

I don't know how my marriage survived it. I was blaming my

husband for not making it better. I feel now that I've crossed a bridge and he hasn't crossed it with me. He tried very hard to support me. I know that at first he felt terribly rejected, like I didn't want him, but I felt isolated and alone, that no one else could help me. I couldn't give him anything. He even resigned from his job and we had to move house again so that we lost a lot of money and we were in terrible financial trouble. He was supportive in a practical way. He always said that I should do what I wanted to do. But somehow I didn't feel that he understood and that he blamed me for it. Now it's his turn to react. I think he's going through a sort of depression. It's still there between us, and I know that now I'm not like I was before I had Daisy.

Daisy seems fine. It used to crack me up when she smiled at me. She was very good considering how I felt about things. I found her difficult because I'd had no dealings at all with a small baby. My mother suffers from anxiety and there was a lot of pressure from her to do it perfectly. As a child myself, I remember I always had to be terribly pretty all the time, and I have lots of memories and images of stuff that happened with her. I used to have a thing about that with Daisy, too. I would get very uptight if my husband dressed her in clothes that didn't match.

My mother has hidden things in her that she doesn't reveal to me. I can't match her perfect image of me. I have always felt that with my mother. Part of the depression must have been due to this. She started off helping me when I was ill, but she couldn't bear to see me fail. I found that the therapist helped me understand all this.

The trouble is that I can't let go, I'm a perfectionist and I used to push myself. My job can't be done on a half-hearted basis, it requires the whole of you. And I can't switch it off, so that if a project comes up, then I want to do it. With Daisy I found that I couldn't be with her, but I couldn't be without her. Now, though, I only work part-time and I've changed.

The thing is, why don't women say anything about motherhood and the effect it has on you? There's a sort of conspiracy of silence between women who have children. I said afterwards to my friends, 'Why didn't you tell me what it would be like?' but they said they thought I'd be able to cope. I was terribly naive and I believed all that natural childbirth stuff.

The classes focused so much on the birth and I was very angry afterwards, because they'd never talked about induction, or problems. We never covered anything like that.

Nobody helps you to understand the complexity of emotions that come with childbirth. And everyone's different. But working and having children, no one ever tells you what it's really like and I'd never experienced emotion on that level before. There's an assumption that you're a Madonna, basking in this maternal glow. Someone actually said, 'oh well, she's one of those creative types, with her histrionics, what do you expect? Why can't she just get on with it like an ordinary person?' Somehow because I could articulate the way I felt, and could sometimes be quite detached about it, and analyse it, they didn't seem to think it was so real.

I think you can be helped quite radically by talking to someone who's been there. You can't do anything to help people in this state without realizing that these feelings, however strange, are very real things. I'm part of a counselling group now, and there are lots of professional women like me. Some of them are in a terrible state.

PND knocked my sense of myself and my personal security. It damaged my faith in my own ability to cope which I'd never challenged before. I was always quite good at problem-solving before, dealing with lots of different things without too many difficulties, but now . . .

With Daisy, I'm always trying to make up to her because of it, always trying to prove that I love her. In a way, although I'm working part-time now, I feel I wasn't really with her during the first year. I felt I was a really bad mother, but I know that she doesn't blame me for it. In a funny way, I feel she understood. Now, though, I sometimes think that if she's having tantrums, or behaving badly, it's because of me.

When you're suffering I think you need to speak to someone who's suffered too. You need something to hold on to as well, so regular contact is important. What helped me was a regular appointment with my therapist. The trouble with PND is that you lose all boundaries. Of course, making that first step is very difficult, it's easier said than done and of course, that's all part of the illness.

You feel so unheard, so invisible. People tell you it doesn't exist, or that it's hormonal, or that women are more prone to mental illness. They see you with a healthy child and they don't understand what you're talking about.

I think, too, that you must acknowledge what stresses there are in your life: what the external factors are like the house, money, job and husband as well as the internal factors. The trouble is that you can't do this at the time. I think you shouldn't stay on your own because it's very hard to take advice when you're feeling that bad. You wonder how you will ever come through it, but I came through it.

It's amazing to me that someone could get that bad and not be noticed. But then, one girl I knew who was going to regular coffee mornings with her friends and used to laugh and joke about how bad she was feeling, was never taken seriously by anyone. She hanged herself. Everyone in her group felt terrible. But I know when you're feeling like that it's hard to believe that anyone else understands.

There are no training courses you can attend on 'Being a Good Mother'. It is something we all have to learn by trial and error. The best piece of advice I was ever given came from a good friend who had two children by the time I was expecting my first. She told me to write off the first six weeks after the birth. She told me to expect nothing, plan nothing and warned that it would take me that long to get used to this creature who was to be entirely dependent on me for its every whim and need.

It comes as quite a shock when your baby cries and people turn to you and ask: 'What's wrong with him then?' and expect you to have the answer. After a while, you will usually know. But it will take you time to recognize his cry above that of other babies, and then to learn that when he cries because he's hungry, it is quite different from the cry he makes when he is tired. No book will be able to help you to tell the difference.

The first few days at home can be particularly hard, too, no matter how much you disliked being in hospital. At least you could devote your time and attention solely to yourself and the baby, without worrying about running a home, cooking and housework, and taking care of other people.

An action plan to ease those first few weeks

● Try to arrange for your mother, your partner, or some close relative or friend to be with you at home for the first week or so. It needs to be someone you feel comfortable and at ease with, someone who is not going to mind if you say you are going up to your room to rest. No matter how well you felt in hospital, you will probably find that once home, you feel worn out very quickly. What you need is someone who is quite happy to get on with the chores for a while, so that you can concentrate on getting used to the baby. It is also a great comfort to have someone there to back you up.

Even if your partner cannot get time off work to be with you, make sure that he realizes just how much work is involved. The only way to do that is to let him know and let him help. Either he can nurse the baby while you get on with something, or he can do some of the routine jobs while you look after the baby.

● Try to decide before the birth whether to breast or bottle feed, who is going to be with you at the birth, and who if anybody is needed to stay at home with other children and how you are going to organize the trip to hospital. Try to get your husband or partner involved as much as possible. He may enjoy this, on the other hand, he may feel it is not for him, so don't force it, but talk to your partner about it and make sure he is aware of what you have decided.

● Talk to your husband or partner about the difference a baby will make to your lives. Talk about the things you do now which you will not be able to do later, or which will be more difficult to do after the birth. Discuss the things you each think you may have to give up or change. If you find it difficult to talk about, each of you should try writing down your own list and then exchange them. Then discuss solutions to each other's difficulties.

● Don't be afraid to read up all you can about the subject, especially about what will happen after the birth and in the first few weeks following and then don't be afraid to ask questions of doctors and nurses at the baby clinic.

- Take advantage of all reasonable offers of help. It doesn't mean that you can't cope or that you are losing control, it simply means that someone is doing you a good turn. Many hospitals offer a babysitting service on the night before a new mother goes home, so that she and her partner can have a couple of hours out. If you don't want to do this, then ask your mother or a good friend to babysit while you go out together, even if it's only for an hour. You may well find it hard to leave your baby, or feel guilty about it. That's only natural, but your baby will come to no harm at all if he is being looked after by someone sensible for a short time. Even if you are breastfeeding, a couple of hours is quite feasible.

- Get to know your health visitor and if you have any worries, talk to her about them. If you're feeling particularly nervous about something, then say so. Many health visitors will give you a phone number where you can reach them at any time and will be quite happy for you to use it. It can be very comforting to know that you have this safety net if ever you need to use it.

  If you don't care for your health visitor, or feel that she isn't very approachable, then do remember that the hospital staff where you gave birth may well be happy to chat to you on the phone if you have any worries. Your doctor, too, will be able to give you advice by phone on any minor problems, and he will be able to tell you whether you need to see him personally.

- There will probably be a baby clinic held on a regular basis in your area where you can take your baby, and apart from an opportunity to meet other mothers with small babies, the health visitor and a doctor will usually be available if you feel you need their advice. There will also be the equipment on hand to weigh the baby if you have any worries on that score.

- Try to get to know at least one other woman who either has a baby the same age as yours, or who perhaps has older children and with whom you can compare notes without feeling that there is a competitive edge to it. There is nothing more off-putting than those situations where young mothers are trying to outdo each other with their babies' achievements.

● However hard and unfamiliar it might feel, try not to worry about anything but the essential housework and chores for the first few weeks. You will have enough to do without polishing the brasses and the 101 other jobs you used to do but which are not vital to the smooth running of your home.

● Being able to have time to yourself is a must, even if it's only the opportunity to put your feet up for an hour while the baby sleeps in the afternoon. Don't allow yourself to be swamped by the baby. The desire to spend time on your own doing something that you enjoy is not wrong and is no reflection on your ability as a mother. If you have hobbies or interests, don't give them up. It might mean that you have to make arrangements for someone to look after the baby, but don't shy away from doing that. It won't do either of you any harm, and will probably do you both good.

● No matter how difficult it might seem, don't give up going out with your baby. The first time you actually manage to get yourself and your baby and the mountain of provisions he seems to need, together, will be comparable to organizing a major expedition, but it does get easier as you get more experienced at it. If you have to use public transport, try to avoid the busiest times, because there is no getting away from it, mothers with babies and children are treated as second class citizens when it comes to getting out and about. If you are going shopping, take notice, for example, of shops such as Mothercare and Boots which have special rooms set aside where you can change or feed your baby.

● Make sure you keep up some sort of social life with your partner. You certainly won't be able to go out as often as you did before you had the baby, but there's no reason why you can't go out once a week or once a fortnight.

● Try not to organize a house move while you still have a tiny baby. Unless it's absolutely unavoidable, you'll have enough to cope with.

● If you have other small children, accept all offers of help with them, but also try and give them their own bit of special time with you alone, so that they don't feel left out, and encourage them to help with the baby. Many mothers are devastated when their older children are not as enthusiastic about new babies as they are. But many mothers make the mistake of talking about a new brother or sister to play with when quite clearly a new baby is not that at all. Far better to be realistic and point out that new babies make a lot of noise, are very demanding and may well be a pain in the neck at first. But they will improve later.

● Most importantly, take care of your own health. Women always tend to put themselves last because they have so many other demands on their time and energy. There are certain things which you must do for yourself, particularly now that you are a mother. You must get enough rest. If you are finding this hard because your baby seems to be awake most of the night and you are becoming more and more exhausted, then you must try and find someone who can take over from you on a regular basis so that at least occasionally you can get a decent night's sleep.

● You must eat properly. You may well be trying to lose weight, or find it difficult to fit meals into this hectic new life, but you must have a sensibly balanced diet to keep yourself going.

● You must get some exercise. No matter how hard you find it, try and keep up with the simple exercises you will have been shown in hospital. They are very quick and easy to do, and although it's difficult to find the time to fit them in, and a chore to do them, they will help you not only physically to get back in trim and to stay that way, but also they will help to keep you fit mentally.

● Make sure you keep up with your routine medical checks such as having a smear test and checking your breasts. And don't imagine that just because you have had a baby you have to put up with all sorts of problems such as disrupted periods. Always check with your doctor if you have any symptoms which are not usual for you.

I've never felt like this before, there must be something wrong with me . . .

When you consider the enormous changes which take place in a woman's body, from the point of conception through the nine months of pregnancy, through childbirth and the return to normal which is usually completed by six weeks after the delivery, it is amazing that any mother gets through it without some problems. The pregnancy has put a huge strain on the body's mechanisms, not just in terms of size but by giving the heart, kidneys and other vital organs much more work to do. Add to that the enormous hormonal changes and there is great potential for physical difficulties.

There are some pathological conditions that can arise from these changes. Sometimes there is a thyroid deficiency. The thyroid gland produces a number of hormones, including one which is responsible for regulating the speed at which the body works. If there is a shortage of this hormone, then the speed slows, and the sufferer finds herself falling asleep at odd times. Other symptoms include dry skin and a change in the condition of the hair which sometimes falls out, and a feeling of being cold. The doctor can check for this problem, if it is suspected, by doing a simple blood test and checking the pulse, which tends to be slow. If a thyroid deficiency is the problem, then it can easily be treated by giving tablets containing the missing hormone. Usually, the body will readjust given time, and the treatment will no longer be needed.

Another common problem is anaemia which leaves a woman feeling exhausted. This often happens after a large loss of blood during the birth and most doctors are on the look-out for this problem. Anaemia too can be diagnosed with a simple blood test and can be corrected by giving iron tablets or injections.

Too tired to cope

Exhaustion can also be caused because a mother is trying to cope with a baby who seems to cry a lot, is difficult to settle or feed, and who does not sleep well. It is a good idea to have the baby checked over in these cases to make sure that all is well and then to get advice on how to cope with the problem. If you are having night after night of constantly broken sleep, then you will quickly become exhausted. After all, breaking regular sleep patterns is a well-established form of torture!

Even if you have had a 'normal' trouble-free birth, it will still take time to get over it. Many women, particularly first-time mothers, find themselves on an emotional 'high' for two or three days afterwards, but this often wears off, leaving them feeling drained and empty. In hospital they will have been the centre of attention with visitors arriving with presents and cards and generally making a fuss. Once home, with the novelty wearing off, a woman is then expected to get on with it and get back to normal quickly. If she already has children, then there is also the expectation that she knows what it's all about, she's done it all before, and she can take a new baby in her stride.

People talk in terms of 'good' babies and 'difficult' babies. The good ones are the ones who sleep a lot and the difficult ones are the wakeful ones. Many new mothers are shocked to discover that their baby is not at all happy to sleep between feeds, let alone through the night. And if that comes on top of another wakeful child it can make for a very stressful situation. Tiredness is the one problem that few parents escape.

Many husbands and partners still regard getting up with the children at night as a woman's responsibility, but just as he needs a good night's sleep to be able to cope with his job, so she needs a good night's sleep to be able to cope with the seven-day-a-week, 24-hours-a-day responsibility of caring for home and family.

If sleeping is a problem, then a mother must have help. If your partner cannot help, or perhaps, he, too, is exhausted, then try and get relatives or friends to help out and take over the night duty on a regular basis so that you can get some unbroken rest. It may not solve the problem completely, but you will be able to cope with the other broken nights much better.

Is there life after babies?

After the long drama of the pregnancy and birth and the excitement of hospital visits and presents, life at home with sole charge of a small baby can come as quite a shock, especially for first-time mothers. Probably the one single word that causes most problems and which you'll hear most often and which almost all the baby books use is 'routine'.

All kinds of regimes will be suggested but the important message coming through loud and clear from almost every source is that babies need routines and will not be happy or thrive without them. So the new mother organizes a routine and tries to stick to it. The first thing that happens is that you realize that a baby's routine organized along these lines does not fit in with ordinary family life. The second thing is that the baby won't stick to it, so the new mother automatically assumes it is her fault, she is not doing things the right way, feels terribly guilty and starts to panic.

The real problem is, of course, that the babies have not read the books, but just like the rest of us, some days they feel like sleeping more than others, some days they feel cross and irritable, some days they are hungry and other days less so, some days they are particularly jolly and feel like being fussed over and entertained. The other thing which is very easy to forget is that they are growing and developing at such a rate that what suits their needs one week, may well have altered the next, and again the following week. Routines are strictly for the mothers' benefit and like any set of rules they are made to be bent and broken.

Another problem which many of the baby experts and books overlook or dismiss in a few words is that of feelings of guilt. This particular emotion seems to me to be the one which no matter what else you might feel, always comes with motherhood.

From the start, mothers are made to feel guilty. Guilty because they didn't always eat sensibly, or had the occasional drink, or did not always feel positive about the baby during pregnancy. Guilty because they had to resort to pain-relief, or a completely high-tech birth. Guilty because they had problems with breast-feeding, or gave it up altogether. Guilty because they used a dummy. Guilty because they resorted to using solids before the baby was three months old. Guilty because they didn't breastfeed for long enough, or breastfed for too long. Guilty because they found looking after small babies boring . . . the list is endless.

I remember a health visitor saying to me after the birth of my first child, when I was worrying about whether or not to go back to work, that whatever I decided I would feel guilty about it, but that as long as I realized this, I could learn to cope with it. It is social pressure that creates the problems in the working/full-time mother dilemma: a woman must make her own choice since there is no right answer as to whether it is the employed or the stay-at-home mothers who should carry the major burden of guilt.

Three things you can do about guilt feelings

● Accept first of all that all babies are different and the way your baby is is different from everyone else's. So what works for one mum will not necessarily work for another.

● You may not have much confidence in your own abilities as a mother, but you are the best one your baby has and you will soon come to know your baby's needs better than anyone else.

● Get yourself organized, rather than worry about a routine. If your baby goes to sleep, and you're feeling tired, then you rest, too. Making your husband's dinner, or doing the ironing or dusting can wait.

A 10-point plan for survival

1. Forget about the housework for a while, or at least stop trying to do it 'properly'. Tidying up can make all the difference, especially if things can be sorted into piles and hidden away behind a sofa. Make it clear to your partner — as nicely as you can — that you really can't cope with cooking an evening meal and looking after the baby, at least for a little while. Don't be tempted to even try being the

perfect wife and mother with a beautiful, neat home, and the ability to turn out a sumptuous dinner party for ten at the drop of a hat.

2. If the sight of baby gear swamping the house gets on your nerves, then try to keep one room completely free of it. At least then you and your partner have somewhere to go where you can relax without being reminded of the mountains of washing that you have suddenly acquired.

3. Be prepared to use all labour-saving devices that you can afford. Don't be too proud to accept hand-me-down baby clothes from friends. The rate at which babies grow means they could never possibly wear out their clothes and the more you have, the less often you will have to do the washing. And certainly in the early weeks, it is quite common for some babies to need a complete change up to six times a day. They have a great talent for throwing up on everything but the bib, and an even greater ability to shoot the contents of their nappies either up their backs or down into the feet of their babygros.

4. If anyone offers help, accept it. If someone offers to come and look after the baby, as long as they're competent and you trust them, accept. If a neighbour or friend offers to do some errands, then let her. And don't be too proud to ask for help if you need a break.

5. Try and keep all the baby things in one place, preferably somewhere with a sink, though not the kitchen. At least then everything is to hand. There is nothing worse than getting a baby half-way through changing its dirty nappy and discovering that the baby wipes are at the other end of the house.

6. Make feeding times — especially night-time ones — as relaxing as possible. Take a drink in a flask to bed with you. Have a book or magazine at hand to read and a light if needed. It is an opportunity for you to rest, too, so make sure you have a comfortable chair.

7. Keep your own meals simple, but don't be tempted to skip them. You must eat regularly and sensibly.

8. Take every opportunity to rest. Don't be afraid to take the phone off the hook, ignore the front door bell and go to bed

when the baby falls asleep. If you know that a friend or neighbour might call and disturb the baby or you, then put a note on the front door asking them not to disturb you, or to call later.

9. Discuss things with your partner, so that there are specific duties which he can do to help you, but make sure you don't exclude him from all contact with the baby.

10. Be prepared to break any or all of these rules if it suits you.

CHAPTER SEVEN
Motherhood changes everything . . .

In days gone by, the coming of motherhood changed everything for a woman. It was generally-accepted practice that women devoted themselves completely to their children, only returning to work in cases of absolute economic necessity or when the children were considered old enough to cope with it. In many cases, motherhood conferred with it a status which lasted for the rest of a woman's life. Once she had children, a mother was never expected to work again.

Women gave up all manner of things to become mothers: interesting, fulfilling jobs, hobbies, holidays, freedoms, and most importantly, time to do things they enjoyed doing. For many women looking after and bringing up children is what they have always wanted, looked forward to, worked for and for many, it is enough. They find that children bring them fulfilment. But many others find that motherhood and the expectations of others are not quite so easy to adjust to. How many times have we all heard women say: 'Nobody ever told me it would be like this . . . I never realized it would be such hard work . . .'.

Sometimes this is the truth. Everyone around a woman has been full of encouragement and promises of how wonderful it will all be with little or no mention of the harsh realities. But many women carried away with the euphoria of getting pregnant and being the centre of attention, take no heed of the warnings given them. It's much nicer to think about and believe in the rosy pictures of happy families and sweet-smelling, gurgling babies than the possibilities of sleepless nights, constant demands and endless washing and feeding.

Adjusting to the changes which parenthood brings is

something which the babycare books tend to skate over. They describe in glowing terms the wonders of a new family and if they do mention problems at all, these are usually dismissed as something which is easily overcome between the happy couple. As most of us know only too well, it just isn't like that. And mothers and fathers who don't live up to the happy, contented image of the perfect family can begin to feel guilty, and can start to blame themselves.

No matter how much a woman wants a baby, no matter how well-prepared, the reality of the situation she finds herself in as a new mother is often not what she expected. As Shirley discovered with the birth of her first baby, despite her husband's warnings, she was completely unprepared for her own feelings about the change a baby made to her life.

Shirley's story

The birth was awful. Everything went wrong. I had an epidural which affected my waterworks and my stomach swelled up and I had to have a catheter. So they kept me in hospital for three weeks and of course, after that long, you don't want to go home because you cling to the security of a hospital. There were lots of younger girls going in and out after 48 hours, and there was me lying with all these tubes, feeling old and incapable. It was the first time in my life that I actually hadn't been able to cope. I had to ask people to show me how to change a nappy, I found it so difficult. I'm not practical and my husband isn't either. He'd already had two children from his first marriage and had made a bad job of it, so he knew what it was like and warned me that it wouldn't be easy. He pulled no punches. Before I got pregnant was one time when we had lots of heart to hearts. He knew it would be difficult and told me he wasn't going to change nappies or be wonderful with the baby. He made me realize that having the baby was my decision.

Once I saw what it actually involved, this tiny creature wanting me, not as I thought on a regular basis, but 24 hours a day. I felt lousy, I felt stitched together with bits of plastic, I had cold sores and looked terrible. And from the beginning Peter was depressed because he saw me being depressed. The nurses and midwives were generally terrific, but there I was with all these young ones coming and going and finding it very easy to adapt to the baby. I'm told Petra was not a bad baby, she was very good. But I said to the nurses that I wanted to feed her regularly, every four hours. I was breastfeeding but I didn't enjoy that either, because I couldn't get on with it. I didn't find it easy. I suspect it was because I wasn't very relaxed; the child wasn't either, so she wasn't taking to it.

And I did *not* get this feeling of bonding. I know it's terrible. She was a very pretty little baby, very good, all these things that I look back on now and think I should have been glad about and enjoyed. But I didn't get any feeling of overwhelming love. This is what really made me feel guilty because I had been told that you would get this amazing glow of satisfaction and love and all that kind of thing and I didn't.

I started to think what had triggered it off. During the pregnancy, Peter had a business trip to Mexico and we'd always managed to go on these trips together, done things together before, and this time they'd found a place for me, but my doctor said I couldn't go. He said that there would be altitude problems and as there were no medical facilities, he didn't advise it. He said anywhere else would have been OK, but not there. I knew he was right and I didn't go, but I resented it. And although the rest of the pregnancy was fine, I suddenly felt things weren't the same any more.

Once the baby was born I found myself thinking: this baby is really going to change me. How am I going to be able to go and do things? I wanted to do everything by the book, and I could see that this thing of feeding every four hours might not work out because she was small and she needed more than some of the others. I had a row with several of the nurses who said I had to demand-feed, and I said no, I didn't want to. I remember seeing a friend demand-feeding and it had horrified me. She would constantly have a child at the breast. She had no time for herself and I thought no, it sounds selfish but I'm not prepared to do that. Then a very nice older sister came to me one day and saw me looking crestfallen and I explained the problem. She was wonderful. She said: it's your baby and whatever you feel you want to do, do it. It'll be better for the baby and for you.' If there'd been more people like that sister around, I don't think I would have had the depression I did.

I was also obsessed with the idea of a routine. That's what

my life had been and because I wanted to get back to work, I thought the way to do it was to get into a routine. In the end the sister had a word with the nurses and she said to me, 'You feed her every four hours and we'll top her up'. And that's what they did. They kept her in the nursery at night which was brilliant for me because it meant I never had any broken nights. I fed her at midnight and they brought her to me again about 6.30 am. But I still didn't like the breastfeeding and she wasn't getting enough, so at five weeks I thought well this is silly, the sister had said that if I preferred the bottle, I should use it. Once I started with the bottle, Petra never looked back. In fact she preferred the bottle. But you see people don't tell you about things like that and I just felt guilty.

I hadn't felt this great surge of affection, and here I was with the bottle. The trouble was I could never bring myself to breastfeed in front of anyone. When my step-children came to visit in hospital — we'd always been close and I adored them — I couldn't bring myself to feed Petra in front of them, so that created a barrier. They suddenly saw me not as a free, coping person. I turned away and hid myself and I felt embarrassed. I couldn't do it in front of the family. I couldn't actually do it in front of my husband. It became a great thing of sneaking off to a bedroom to do it furtively. So it became a performance instead of a nice, natural thing. Peter didn't feel very easy about it because I didn't. It was really total chaos.

In hospital I could also see all these younger dads and younger brothers and sisters all coming in and rushing up to the hospital beds. You know how you have this rosy glow with the little three-year-old coming to see the baby. I didn't have any of that. In fact Peter's daughter Lucy who was 16 — a difficult age anyway, especially when her parents were divorced — was very depressed about it. Her nose had been put out of joint. She was very close to her father and had it been a boy, I think she would have been OK, but she actually hated the baby. It's fine now, they adore each other, but for the first year, she hated Petra. She wasn't very verbal about it. She didn't come into the hospital and create, but you could see her face was just rigid. There was this little figure hovering at the end of the bed. Peter always hovered too because he didn't know if I'd be in a heap of tears. In contrast to that were these other happy families all round us.

I hadn't really organized myself. I was relying on a neighbour who had offered to help me out. I thought it would be better to have someone I knew looking after the baby rather than getting involved with childminders in the abstract. But it really didn't work because she wouldn't take any payment. I didn't have my Mum with me then and I would always say to a woman that I think Mum is one of the best people you can have around you when you've had a baby. But mine lived up north and I didn't want to involve her. I didn't want her to see me not coping, for which she will never forgive me. What I should have done was to get her down as soon as I came out of hospital.

When I came home I felt terribly isolated. I'd lived in the village and loved it, but I used to go up to town and work five days a week. I knew nobody except this very kind neighbour, so there was this awful isolation, coupled with ineptitude at breastfeeding and I just found that my life revolved around every four-hour feed. The child did sleep in between, and I'd thought I'd do all sorts of things but I felt knackered. All I could do was catch up on sleep. I remember thinking, well, this is what my life's going to be like from now on: absolutely revolving around this tiny little mite: of course, resentment sets in. She must have sensed that I was unhappy because she wasn't as happy as she should have been. It was horrific. I had one friend who had her baby shortly after I did and we used to talk on the phone. I think if she hadn't felt the same way as I did, I would have gone mad, or at least I would have leapt on a train to my mum's.

Peter didn't know what to do about it. I felt this total resentment because he was able to carry on as normal, coming back each night and thinking he was helping by telling me all about what had gone on at work. This was exactly what I couldn't stand. But stupidly, instead of thinking — now who can I talk to about this (I had lots of friends who would have helped), I didn't want anybody to know.

My doctor was an elderly gent who looked after me very well physically, and in fact I got better rather quickly, but he never asked me how I felt. The only person I mentioned it to was this friend on the phone. We didn't know what to do. We were only 25 miles apart and we couldn't help each other. In the end she asked what were we going to do and I decided to start some work.

I left Petra with this very kind neighbour, but since she wouldn't take any money, I felt guilty giving Petra to her for two days on the trot. But it wasn't enough and I couldn't get my teeth into anything. I couldn't ever fit anything in around Petra, because I found her totally time-consuming. In the end my mum came down to stay after about eight weeks (she'd been looking after my father who was ill) and she realized straight away what was wrong. She was horrified at the state I was in, and said I must get someone to look after the baby properly and do more work. But I felt so despondent, I didn't see how I could do it. She did tell me that this four-hourly thing would pass, and in the meantime not to worry too much and to use my lovely neighbour.

But she came down again two months later and found me in the same awful mess. I was weeping all the time. I would actually sit on the floor, I didn't know what to do. It was despair. I used to bang my hands on the floor because I didn't know what to do. I knew that when the child was sleeping it was only for X number of hours. She wasn't a naughty baby, but I just had no time. I couldn't do anything. The house was a mess. I'd never been very good at housework anyway, and I felt totally imprisoned. If Petra did cry, I had no patience. I used to shake her. I understand about baby battering. Many a time, I would shake her; I had to walk away sometimes because I knew if I didn't I would do something awful. I used to shout at her: 'Shut up, you little bitch'. It wasn't the child's fault, she was very good.

It annoyed me that I couldn't do these basic chores that other people found so easy. For the first time in my life I was a dunce — after doing well at school, at a job — suddenly here I was at 33 and I couldn't do it. It was terrible, and unfortunately there was nobody there to say that it didn't matter. I wanted desperately to be as capable at motherhood as I had been at my job. I felt terrible. I didn't want to get up in the morning. Sunday was the same as Monday, Saturday the same as Wednesday. I'd always looked forward to weekends, but they weren't special any more. I still had to feed the little brat every four hours. I wanted to be so ill that people would find me and I'd be taken back into hospital, relieved of the child. I wanted to be found out, so that everybody would know and then somehow everything would be put right.

In a funny way, I did have a routine with her. When the four-hourly thing stopped, then she would always have a sleep morning and afternoon. She went to bed at seven, and never broke my night's sleep. But it was absolutely not doing me any good because I wasn't relaxed at all. I couldn't do anything because I was too frightened. You know how you see people wrap their babies up and take them out, I just couldn't do it. People had told me about a group of young mums in the village hall and said I ought to go down there. I couldn't bear it because I worried about what I would do if she woke up, instead of just thinking well if she wakes up, so what.

I wouldn't go anywhere, there always seemed to me to be so much paraphernalia. I remember once Peter came home from work and said he wanted to go to York on business and he wanted me to come with him. And I said well, what about Petra, and he said, 'Bring her.' I fell in a heap, I couldn't think about it. Then the nice neighbour said to me, 'Look, this is his way of trying to help. You've got to do it. If you lose this, you may well lose him.' She was right, and she helped me get it together. I took everything but the kitchen sink, and the whole trip was a disaster and I hated every minute of it. That was the only time we ever did anything like that until Petra was a lot older.

When she was five months old, two things happened which I think were the turning point. A woman in the village — she wasn't even a friend at that time — who I'd seen, always looking wonderful, beautifully made up, hair, the lot; she had a baby, and I thought always had things organized and she saw me one day and just said, you look so unhappy, why don't you get a cleaning lady? I told poor Peter who was distraught by this time and didn't know what to do about me, and he said 'Please get a cleaning lady and if you want to get a childminder, please get a childminder.' But we were both worried about that, because she was so small and she had bad colic and was underweight, so we decided to leave it for three or four months and then see.

The cleaning lady came and was terrific, very practical and at least it meant I didn't have to fiddle around the house and I only had Petra to consider. She showed me how to do a nappy. It doesn't have to be perfect, she told me, it doesn't matter. And if she cries, as long as it's not a piercing cry, then leave her, it won't do any harm for half an hour. And she said I shouldn't worry about the house looking untidy because that's the way it would be from now on with a child about. She was very basic and nobody had ever said these things to me before.

Then the neighbour started to take the baby a couple of days at a time, and I could manage bits of work and I realized it was good. Then my mum came down again and saw that I still wasn't really happy, still the floods of tears, still this isolation. I hadn't got on with the people in the village — they were lovely, nothing against them — but they were young mums, dying to give up work and have a baby and they couldn't understand that I wasn't supremely happy. I'd never told them what my job was, because I didn't want to sound clever, but one day someone asked me, and I told them, and the whole group I was with just walked off. Peter reckons I built it out of all proportion, but I don't think so. I just think they couldn't handle it. They didn't know how to talk to me, what to say, I just didn't get on with them. I had nothing in common. I didn't go down to the group in the village hall because I didn't want to talk about the price of nappies. I felt terrible, because Peter said I should give them a chance, because I'd have to be around them with school and everything. But they didn't give me a chance. There was no meeting ground. Then another very kind woman whose husband works in the same job as us, when she saw I was here with a small baby, she leapt on me. She was very kind and kept inviting me to coffee mornings. Peter said just go to one, so I did and I couldn't believe it, it was so awful. I just couldn't become part of this village thing. I didn't want to. Why should I?

Then the nice girl who'd got me the cleaning lady said if I needed someone to look after Petra more often, then she might know of someone who'd be interested. Mum came down to look after Petra then, while Peter and I went off for four days' holiday. She said that she thought I needed to work more than two days and why didn't I get someone and pay them for looking after the baby. So this wonderful lady called Mary came. She spent three weeks coming in and getting to know Petra and she was marvellous. And really the minute I started doing three days' regular work with the baby off my hands — on those days I didn't want to see her at all — it was absolutely wonderful and the two days with Petra didn't seem so bad at all. I had a lot more patience, and I even went down to the

village group once or twice for Petra's sake. That wasn't quite
as bad either.

When I began to find it easier, of course Peter found it easier.
I don't think I realized it was post-natal depression until she was
about nine months old and I read a book about organizing
yourself with a new baby. The authors said that organization
was the way to beat the baby blues, so that the baby didn't
swamp you. I suddenly thought, that is exactly what has
happened to me. I hadn't organized myself properly.

I'd always organized everything else. I was a furious list-
maker — at the beginning of every day I have my list. I think
what threw me was the actual birth, the knowledge that the
little person who was now here was completely dependent on
me. It's very different being on the outside of that from being
on the inside. I should have been more organized, for instance,
instead of depending on the neighbour (wonderful though she
was) it made me feel dreadful, so beholden because she wasn't
getting paid. That was my mistake. I think if I'd had Mary from
say three or four months, things would have been a lot
different. It was probably a year before I really got myself sorted
out and on top of it. But Mary was probably the real turning
point, though it did take me a few months of getting over that
guilt thing of enjoying the freedom. I was working damned
hard for it; it took some organizing, getting up at 6.30 am to
make sure everything was there for the childminder. But that
was better for me. Somehow it didn't seem as awesome as
waking up at 7.30 am and knowing that I'd be here all day, and
what was I going to do.

On reflection now, I don't think my relationship with Petra
has suffered, because if anything I've almost over-
compensated and I do think, and this is a cliché, that it's a
matter of quality time. At one point I did think that she was
going to love Mary more than me. When she was about 1½
years old you could see the delight on her face when Mary
came. I think it was because Mary was calm, placid, middle-
aged, warm, with brown cheeks and never ruffled at anything,
whereas Mummy was a bit fraught. There was this tiny period
(although I knew that I'd never give up my work) when I
thought that my reward for all this would be that the child
would turn to her childminder or whoever before she would
turn to me. But it was short-lived because Mary used to talk to

me about it; she made me feel much better because she would always reassure me that this wouldn't happen, that she would never take my place with Petra. She was a very wise lady.

As Petra got older I began to take more interest anyway. The awful restraint of those regular feeds had gone and on my two days off, the time I gave her was jam-packed full of me. I think — and don't laugh — I actually didn't love Petra from birth. I didn't want her at all. Having had this much-wanted child, I kept thinking what it was like before she was there. So I was negating her. I thought it was nicer when she wasn't around. We used to go on these little holidays for three or four days, just Peter and I (that was my mum again saying we should go and she would come and look after Petra) and I jumped on the plane. I didn't miss her, I loved it. It was being a couple again. Once you have a child you aren't a couple any more and I found it very difficult to adapt from being lovers, to being a family. I used to feel ill at ease with baby, Peter and I. It was very silly because it's totally natural and wonderful, and now I just can't bear the thought of her not being there. I think I fell in love with Petra when she was about two. Peter would hate me saying this because he thinks I got it out of all perspective, but I think it's true.

When she was two we went away to Venice and we both sat on the bed in this hotel room and we became aware after an hour that we'd done nothing but talk about her. I suddenly said: 'Oh, Peter, I do love her', and I'd never said that before. I'd never said I loved my child. Isn't that dreadful? I realized what I'd done, and I used to lie awake at night sometimes, thinking don't punish me, God, by taking away that child. I realize how wicked I've been, I still do it now. I think, do anything, let it happen to me, or Peter, or some other member of the family, but not Petra. I feel there's so much to make up for. I suppose I feel I missed out. And I think if I'd gone about it the right way I could have had a lot more out of those early months.

All these other mums looked at me aghast when they heard I'd gone back to work. One of them actually used the word 'abandon'. Mary told me not to worry, she said they were just jealous, and I think there's something in that. They were horrified when we'd gone off on our little holidays, leaving Petra behind. But the minute they could get their kids into playschool, they didn't ease them in with half a day to start with, it was straight in five mornings a week at 2½. They couldn't wait to get rid of them. And you see them in the street, with two or three and they don't talk to them, the only things they ever say are to shout or snap at them, followed by a smack. Over the years, as I've seen these women I used to think were wonderful mothers, mothers I couldn't possibly emulate, and you go in their houses which are pigsties, with the children stuck in the corner in front of the television with a bar of chocolate. That's the way they cope. You hear them say things like 'I just love babies', and they've got a little two-year-old listening. Well, aren't they babies? And they say things like, 'Aren't you glad you've got her off your hands?' I don't want my child ever 'off my hands'. So I think now, it's a pity I didn't know all this before, I would have coped better.

I've never wanted any more than one child. But after my experience, no way would I go through that again. Fortunately Petra has got her step-brother and sister and they're very close. I sometimes think she's a very self-contained child and wonder whether that stems from her early childhood. I was never very good at those baby games.

At the time I worried about my career, but now I wouldn't ever entertain a full-time executive job, because I think there's a bit more to life. You'd turn around at 50 and what have you got then? A child gone, and you've missed it all. But when will people realize that motherhood is an important job? Isn't it demeaned? I remember on my 'mummy' days in jeans and an anorak I didn't want anyone to see me pushing the pushchair. I once went up to London with her and was ignored by porters; no one tried to help me, I was completely ignored. The following day, in my business suit with a briefcase, it was completely different. I said to Peter: 'Do you wonder why women get depressed? You've never had to put up with that.' You begin to be a drudge when you're treated like that. Now I make a point of dressing up to go to school and collect Petra.

I feel very strongly that women have got to be told that it can happen the way it happened to me. They should be told about post-natal depression. That this glorious fulfilment thing happens for some — yes — but not all. Peter and I very nearly didn't survive it. I thought we would have divorced at the end of that first year. We didn't communicate at all. His first wife had done the lot and here he was with a non-coping second wife, ten years younger, who tried to pretend everything was all right, but crying all the time. I've often said that if I'd had the guts, if I'd had the money, if I'd been able to drive a car, I would have gone . . ..

Making choices

Women can be their own worst enemies. I remember when I had my first baby and returned to a job I loved after three months, I was the only working mother on the small modern estate where we lived. On several occasions I was made to feel like an outcast, and several women made it quite clear that as I was not doing the job of being a mother 'properly', then I certainly was not eligible for membership of their exclusive little group of new mothers. And the fact of my working was used as a cause for almost anything that happened to us as a family, but particularly to my children. If they behaved badly, if they were ill, if they were slow at any stage of their development, it was because their mother abandoned them and went out to work. When I first went up to the school gates, because I was not there every day, many of the women who were my neighbours could barely bring themselves to speak to me. They certainly did not allow me into their circle.

On the other hand, some working mothers can be just as destructive. They talk about how being 'just a mother' is not enough for them. I know of several women who have returned to work within days of their child's birth with the express intention of not becoming too attached to the baby. Is it any wonder that new mothers find themselves in the middle of an emotional minefield? And that is without the practical complications of sorting out adequate childcare arrangements if and when you do decide to return to work.

No one can know how the birth of a child will affect them emotionally. And yet many women make momentous decisions during their pregnancy. They may decide to give up work or to go back to work and then find that once the baby has arrived they feel quite differently. And for a lot of women it takes time and patience to arrive at what is usually a compromise between their own needs, those of their baby, and the economic reality of their particular family situation. Post-natal depression in one form or another is what happens to very many women in the meantime.

CHAPTER EIGHT
Finding a way out of a silent illness

The next case history illustrates just how insidious post-natal depression can be. Nancy is a health visitor and, on her own admission, her work should have given her an insight into the problems she faced. When she was feeling at her most depressed, she still continued to work alongside other health professionals and managed to hide her illness from those around her. Small wonder, then, that so many women manage to do the same thing.

Nancy's story

It was my first pregnancy, totally uncomplicated, and I felt wonderful. In fact, I felt so good that I'd done all sorts of things right at the end that most people at that stage wouldn't normally do. I was a health visitor, so I'd seen and heard enough about nasty deliveries to know I wanted to avoid that, and I'd decided to have an epidural. According to my notes it was a normal delivery, quite straightforward, but I felt it was far from that: for me it was gruesome.

I suppose it was one of the complications of knowing too much, but I was perfectly happy at home in the early stages of labour, so I left it as long as possible before going into hospital. When I got there I was already 5 cms dilated and they said I was too far gone for an epidural, that the baby would be here quite soon. That knocked my confidence. Then a bit later the baby's heartbeat went a couple of times and I was threatened with forceps. They talk about that unbearable urge to push, well, I never had that. They say the second stage is much better than first because it's more positive. But for me it was much worse. I was shattered. I just thought I've got to force myself to push to avoid the forceps. I managed without them in the end, but I did need an episiotomy and the whole thing took much longer than they said it would.

For the first 24 hours I was physically and emotionally flattened. I couldn't even get out of bed. Until you're actually in there yourself, you don't know what it's going to be like. I thought I'd been fairly well prepared. One of the pitfalls of having worked with most of the people in the unit was that they took it for granted that here was somebody who knew all about it. So when they brought her to me for the first feed, nobody came to help me. They just left me to it and I remember looking down at her and thinking it's lucky for both of us that I know a bit about it. After that first 24 hours, I felt OK for the rest of my stay in hospital. I was in for six days, and the baby fed well and I coped well. It was obvious that having worked with babies I had the confidence when handling her. I remember people commented on that. I expected to get the 'blues' at about three or four days, but I didn't.

Six weeks after she was born we had some friends to stay and I went shopping with my friend. I was then a whole stone lighter than I had been before I was pregnant. I was delighted at the time, but I later wondered whether it wasn't related in some way. It was too great a weight loss.

Three months later, by Christmas, I was feeling foul, though I don't have a very clear memory of those months. I used to spend hours just sitting in a chair doing nothing. I had no energy, no interest, no nothing. I used to go back to bed after the early morning feed and just stay there until she woke up again. At about five in the afternoon, I used to think, my husband will be home soon, I've got to do something. But all I did was look after her and load the washing machine. I didn't touch the housework.

People would invite me out for lunch, and I would always ring at the last minute and cancel. Because we live in an isolated place, people don't just drop in and we have no family nearby, so if ever I did see anybody it was always by arrangement and I could put on a good show. It went on for months like that. Then in the spring I was asked to do a baby clinic standing in for one of the other health visitors. I spent the afternoon confidently coping with all the other mothers and their babies, and then I was weeping and wailing all the way home. I used to take my child to all the baby clinics and sit there looking at all the other mothers thinking in a very detached way: do they feel the way I do or are they all as happy as they seem? If they're not then they're putting on a better show than me.

It was like a big black cloud hanging over me. I felt totally alienated from everybody. My husband knew that something was very wrong because I would collapse in floods of tears every evening, but we thought it was just something to do with having a first baby and we didn't look any further than that. An illness like PND never crossed my mind. Yes, I'd come across it myself before obviously, but the peculiar thing was it never occurred to me that I had it.

A couple of times, I remember, when she was still small enough to go in the carrycot on the back seat of the car, I drove to a local beauty spot and just sat there thinking about driving off the cliff into the sea. I imagined what it would be like to drown. I wondered whether or not I would take her with me, or whether I would put her out on the side of the road. I wondered how long it would take me to drown. At home sometimes I would sit and plan my escape. I wanted to go as far away as possible. I had a friend in Ireland and for some reason that seemed the best place to go. I wondered would I take the baby or would I leave her in the house but escape just before my husband came home from work, so that she wouldn't be on her own for too long. As for sleeping, I just couldn't get enough of it. I wanted to be left alone in my bed to die.

So we staggered along, I must have been absolutely foul to live with. My husband knew something was wrong, but this illness puts up such a barrier. I couldn't say anything to him. If he asked me what was wrong, I just used to dissolve in tears and run out of the room. Then May came and the christening and I remember the day before thinking I couldn't do it, I couldn't possibly get everything ready. Somehow we muddled through.

I gradually began to get better after that. I was doing more clinics, filling in for holidays, and by September I must have been better, because suddenly I had this pre-menstrual 'crash'.

For 48 hours just before my period, the black cloud came back. This went on for three months, just before every period, and I suddenly worked out what was happening. I went to my doctor then and told him I thought I'd been suffering from post-natal depression and when I described the symptoms he agreed. I made sure he put it down in my notes for the next pregnancy, because I knew I'd be more susceptible.

It didn't put me off having a baby, because having realized what it was, I made sure everyone knew about it. The people I worked with were absolutely horrified because they just hadn't seen it. They felt useless, but once I'd pinpointed it I felt much better. There's nothing worse than not knowing what's happening to you. The only way they could have picked it up would have been if there had been spot visits. But I didn't have any of those, I suppose partly because of who I was, they thought I didn't need them.

I'd always had a regular 28-day-cycle before and never had any PMS, but all that had suddenly changed. When I was 16 weeks pregnant with my second child, I was sent to a psychiatrist and we talked about the hormonal side of it all. I was fine during the pregnancy except that I was a lot more uncomfortable and I didn't feel so well, especially at the end. There were no complications and the birth was much better, he just popped out after I'd had the sort of contractions where I wanted to push.

The psychiatrist came to see me during that first week for a chat and at the end of it was going to sign me off. I had to insist that I saw him again. I was a bit weepy for the first fortnight and I did think, oh no, here we go again, but that passed, and after six weeks I saw him again and I was feeling fine and I was discharged. Despite the fact that we were all ill when I first came out of hospital with him, which couldn't have helped, the difference in the way I felt after him, compared to my daughter, was quite remarkable. After just a few weeks I felt normal.

Again, after my second baby, once my periods restarted, I got this complete despair 48 hours before my period, and occasionally I've felt down right in the middle of the cycle. I've been fascinated to read about Dr Dalton's work. I've had no treatment, though I think that my hormones have altered the pigment in my face. I've got lots of blotches that I never had before.

I have a very different outlook now. I feel the whole thing just isn't talked about enough. There ought to be much more information available. When I went to see my obstetrician during the second pregnancy and we talked about my seeing a psychiatrist, he said he supposed I'd like to go privately and that he wouldn't put it in my notes. I told him that wasn't the point. I wanted it in my notes, so that if it happened again, it would be picked up. It shouldn't be hidden away. It's that kind of attitude that stops anything being done. When I told my colleagues, they wanted to know all about it — I think they found it quite an eye-opener.

We've got a local support group going on a mum-to-mum basis now and we've got quite a few cases, some quite bad ones. But when Dr Dalton came down to this area to talk about her work, all the GPs round here had been notified but just two turned up out of over a hundred. Again when we organized a study day on the subject, only one bothered to come.

After training as a health visitor, I was one of those who didn't think you needed to have a baby yourself to be able to do the job well. Now I'm not so sure. It puts a very different light on things. You understand so many little things far better. I must have been useless before when attempting to cope with it. I remember coming across women with PND and thinking that the doctor was treating it, so it wasn't something I had to worry about. I can't have been much help. I look forward to going back to work now, I think I'll get much more out of it and be better at it.

My advice to people dealing with new mothers who don't seem to be well, though it might sound a bit hard, is not to believe a word they say. You need time and a good relationship with the mother and you need to visit her regularly at home to see if she's coping. You can pick up a lot that way.

Openness and honesty are the important things. You have to accept that PND is a short-lived thing and you will come out of it a sane, normal person. Now when I talk to friends and other women and I tell them about my experience, it's amazing what they will admit to. I would like a third baby, but I've said to my husband that if I become ill again, he's got to get me to a doctor. No matter how much I deny it, he must not take any notice. I'm not prepared to risk going through that again.

Making the decision to become a mother

Motherhood is very different from how it was for most of our mothers. Many women these days have had a comfortable lifestyle, become settled in a pleasant house and have enjoyed a certain amount of freedom before deciding to have a child. For most, having a baby has been part of their partnership plan, or it has crept up on them almost as an overwhelming biological urge.

The majority of women have to face a change of status on becoming a mother. As a society we have a tendency to want to keep mothers and children separate from the so-called 'productive' members. It comes as a shock to realize that walking down the street with a pram, you are seen in a completely different light from the woman walking down the street with a briefcase in hand. With a child in tow, you are very often labelled as somebody's mother, not as a person in your own right. Women also often find that after being the centre of attention for nine months during their pregnancy, relatives and friends then focus all the attention on the child. Many women unconsciously go along with this judgement of themselves as somehow less important. Many times, you can see beautifully turned out children being pushed in a pram by women who have quite obviously not taken any trouble at all with their own appearance.

Motherhood is not easy, but it's very difficult to admit that. It's even harder to own up to the fact that you do not enjoy it or like it much either. And it can be very difficult for those who made a definite decision during pregnancy, either to give up work, or to go back to it, to admit after the birth of their baby that they want to change their minds. If at all possible, it is much better to leave the situation open. Many employers these days are amenable to this.

For those mothers who decide to return to work, there is then the question of childcare. Although the situation is slowly beginning to improve, it is still difficult to decide which method is right for you. Few women these days have the luxury of having either their mother or other close family nearby to help and support them. Whether you choose a childminder, a nanny, a place in a nursery or whatever, it is your decision, and one you must be happy with.

One of the most difficult things to cope with, after the birth of a first child particularly, is the strength of emotions which women feel for their child. This can range from a passionate love-at-first-sight rush of feelings (for the lucky few) through to an enormous weight of responsibility for the small creature you have just produced. I always remember that advice given by my wonderful health visitor after the birth of my own first child when I was thinking about going back to work. She warned me that I would feel guilty, no matter what my final decision was, but that this was very normal and nothing to worry about. Guilt seems to be tied up with motherhood in an inextricable way, and all the more so for working mothers. They feel guilty because they are leaving their children and guilty again because they are enjoying their work.

For stay-at-home mothers there is often another set of pressures. Regular visits to the baby clinic or a mother-and-toddler group can be a source of difficulty for some mothers. Inevitably it seems, these occasions turn into an opportunity to make comparisons. For a woman who is not feeling completely on top of her new situation it can be very disturbing and threatening. Very often women who are feeling depressed do not turn up for this very reason. The talk of babies feeding well, sleeping through the night, smiling, crawling, sitting up, walking and all the other developmental milestones in a baby's life can be very worrying. And of course, the presence of all those coping, happy mothers often confirms a depressed mother's worst fears — she feels isolated and alone because she is not like all the rest.

Older mothers

I would like to make a special mention of older mothers and also to include in this group women who have perhaps had problems conceiving a child. For them the feelings of depression may be greater. After all, haven't they waited such a long time, or tried so hard and gone through so much to produce a baby? And aren't they especially lucky to have been successful? For them the birth of the baby may be the culmination of years of effort, hopes and fears.

So for those women the feelings of inadequacy and depression, not to mention the guilt, can be particularly upsetting. Some older women who have maybe held down a difficult job or career, suddenly find that a new baby brings them face to face with a situation they cannot handle. For the first time, they feel out of control, unable to cope, desperately tired. This is quite common.

Adoptive mothers and single mothers, too, face particular problems. Here is Pauline's story, which like all the others in this book, has a happy ending. Pauline's son is now 15, a bright, happy teenager who is doing well at school and who has a very good relationship with his mother. Pauline remembers well the awfulness of her post-natal depression, but her son has no idea that his babyhood was any different from any other child's.

Pauline's story

I had a complicated medical problem after the birth which led to an operation about 10 days later and meant that I couldn't get out of hospital for a long time. But just before they sent me home, I was getting very fed up so they let me go out into the street for a walk. I was all on my own and had a complete panic attack. It was the first time it had ever happened. I remember being stranded on a traffic island, not knowing which way to go and I could hardly get back to the hospital on my own.

From the beginning I didn't feel anything about the baby — a total blank — I had no maternal feelings towards him, not even a feeling of friendliness. And yet at the same time I had this peculiar feeling of attachment. He was like part of my own body. It wasn't love. I got very upset when he cried, it was like` it was happening to me. I couldn't separate myself from him. When he screamed, I screamed. I felt he was angry with me. Everything was him and me. It was like we were stuck in this bottle together. It was almost as if I hadn't given birth and he was still part of me. I suppose I felt then like most people feel when they are pregnant.

My husband was desperately keen for a baby, though I wasn't so sure. Our relationship was a bit rocky, but in the end we were both looking forward to it. My husband was mad about him which made me feel worse. There were feelings of complete uninterest punctuated by feelings of intense love and affection but at inappropriate times. When I was doing things like ironing his nighties, I would be in floods of tears because they were so small and sweet.

I was terribly sensitive to criticism. People only had to say something like: 'It's a pity he hasn't got more hair', or 'do you think he's warm enough?' or worse still: 'is he hungry?' I felt so inadequate and I'd get absolutely furious with them. And when people said things like: 'aren't you proud of him?' or 'what a clever girl you are', I used to think what do you mean? I felt a terrible fraud, not at all clever, as if I were pretending to be clever. Then I'd hate them and think: why are you trying to do this to me?

Then there was the endless tiredness. I was crying a lot of the time. Sex was terribly painful. Having the baby had been a way of mending our relationship, but it became obvious that we were breaking up. I didn't like to think of the baby having any other family except me and mine. I couldn't bear his grandmother being interested in him, because he was mine. I thought they would steal him from me.

My self-confidence was non-existent. I couldn't accept help, because I couldn't admit that he could do without me, even for an hour. It made me feel even more useless. I thought there's no point in my being here. It was an admission of inability. I could see things only in black and white.

On the one hand I was very protective. I was going to look after him for life but I had feelings of absolute hatred, too. I used to imagine him falling out of his chair, just bouncing out and I'd get feelings of pleasure from that. It was this terrible thing of taking responsibility for everything that happened to him, but getting a secret pleasure from everything that made him miserable.

I had terrible fantasies and dreams. I dreamt of maiming him and gouging his eyes out. The worst dream was hearing him crying and picking him up and kissing and cuddling him and being very sweet to him, then when I put him down in his cot as I watched he became covered in terrible bruises and marks as if I had actually been hitting him. What I was really doing was punching, kicking, hitting him. I woke up feeling really weird after that dream.

I did try to talk to one or two people about it and I went down to the local mother and baby group. But no one understood what I was saying. In fact they'd get up and move away as if I had the plague. I suppose you can understand it in a way, someone saying all these strange things to them. Some would say, yes, isn't it awful trying to cope with a new baby, but no one understood the depth of feeling.

I went to my GP but he asked if I'd like to have the baby taken into care. I think the idea behind it was to give me a break — because I was on my own by then — but I don't think he put it quite the right way and I was horrified. He gave me anti-depressants, but he didn't suggest counselling. At one stage I went to a psychotherapist, but only once. He told me I wasn't holding the baby properly. He said that I held him away from me, rather than close to me, and that was because I was trying to push the baby away. Remarks like that really didn't help at all. It's what I hated about them. It's probably something we all do, instead of someone just saying to me: don't worry, it's all right, they tried making suggestions all the time. The health visitor kept suggesting ways to improve things, try this or that, out of the best possible motives. They give you false hopes because when you try everything and it doesn't work, you feel in the wrong. I just wished someone had said it was fine and not to worry.

He was a very clingy baby and I thought that was my fault. I breastfed him although I didn't particularly like it. Then he was a late weaner, not until he was two, and that made me feel guilty. It set me apart from people and I was criticized for it, so I felt worse and worse. He cried and cried, it seemed to me all day. At the same time I was desperately unable to take any action to stop him. I was too depressed. I was terribly lonely on my own as well. It was difficult to see where one problem ended and another began. To be depressed when you've got someone around is rather different from being depressed all on your own. At least you feel as if someone is around taking care of things. I felt I needed someone to look after me. My husband didn't seem to think there was anything wrong with me at all.

I used to have to go out a lot. It was the only place I felt safe. I would go out in the street and I felt that all the people around me were helping in some way. The baby was better, too. He was very taken with everyone else's activities. When we went to other people's houses, they always seemed better equipped for babies than mine. I didn't have a room decorated especially with elephants and that sort of thing. I never felt I was doing it right. I remember these houses smelling of talcum powder and that smell always made me feel better.

I was convinced he was going to suffer and I wanted to do so well by him. I was setting myself impossible standards. I suppose it went back to my own childhood. I desperately wanted to give him what I didn't have. It was crucial to his well-being. I remember once having this incredible flashback, right to when I was a baby. I was standing in my cot wearing a little Viyella nightdress — I could feel the material in my little hands — and I was screaming and screaming, but no one came.

When I had post-natal depression, my own mother was too depressed herself at the time to help. She was trying to commit suicide. My stepmother was very good, marvellous with the baby and I never felt jealous with her. It would have helped to have a mother like her. She was a terrific support, without her I don't know what I would have done. I had one friend, too, who was just as obsessive as me about getting things right. She was a great help, too.

I suppose the first three years were the worst. But once he started to go to nursery school at about three, the fantasies stopped and that was a great relief. I'd never told anyone about them because I was afraid the men in white coats would take me away. Now I know it's quite a familiar symptom and I've talked to people since who've had them.

No one ever mentioned post-natal depression to me. It gradually dawned on me much later what it was, but I would have been terribly relieved at the time to know what it was. The problem with PND, I think, is that you manage to put on such a good front. And in many ways everyone else can see your love and concern for the child — in fact, I remember once a friend saying to me when I was talking about my feelings that it was quite obvious I loved the baby very much — but it's cut off from you. It's very bizarre, you cut yourself off from yourself. I remember reading a book by some psychologists about how parents treat their children. Some of the things in there were so appalling it made me feel a lot better. It gave me more confidence in myself as a mother. You imagine that everyone else is bonding and blooming, and you're the only one who's not . . .

Post-natal depression is in many ways a silent illness. To the outsider there are few signs and symptoms, particularly if you do not know the sufferer well. It is an isolating illness and one which is all the more difficult to deal with because of that. Women who are ill with PND do not think of themselves as ill in the conventional sense. They see themselves as inadequate, poor mothers, with an inability to cope. Several of the mothers I spoke to said that having suffered themselves they could often spot it in others and would make a point of speaking to women they thought were going through it. In Shirley's story, for example, the neighbour who approached her and commented on how unhappy she was had obviously spotted something which family, friends, professionals had missed. Many women told me that the only people who really understood them were others who had been through it, too. All agree that whatever other treatment might be offered, talking through feelings with someone who understood was an enormous help.

Very many of the women I spoke to had never had any form of treatment, but had gradually got better themselves. Perhaps the first stage on the road to recovery was the realization that this was an illness, even when no one else supported the idea. It seems almost incredible that even the professionals themselves, nurses and health visitors, can suffer from PND and neither they nor the people around them realize it.

A final check list of ideas to help you combat PND

1. Find someone sympathetic to talk to. Try family and friends, your doctor, a social worker, the health visitor or contact one of the voluntary organizations mentioned. It cannot be stressed enough that this is a serious illness, but it is one you will recover from. It can help a great deal if someone you trust can convince you of that. Several of the mothers I spoke to made the point that when they tried to talk about

how they felt to people who had not suffered from PND, there was a complete lack of understanding. This is even more the case when it comes to revealing the strange dreams and fantasies which are often a symptom of the illness. One mother said that people were horrified by what she told them. It was only when she started describing her thoughts to a fellow PND sufferer that she got a sympathetic reaction.

2. Do not be afraid to take the drug treatment offered by your GP. It will not solve all your problems and it is unlikely to be the total remedy to the problem, but it can often help by lifting your mood sufficiently to enable you to talk to someone. There has been so much publicity about tranquillizers and anti-depressants that many people have become afraid to use them at all. Not all these drugs by any means are addictive and if used sensibly over a short period of time, they can be a great help. If you are in doubt, ask your doctor exactly what you are taking, what the side effects are, and whether they are addictive. Explain your fears. If you are not satisfied with the answer you get, then ask to see someone else, a consultant, a therapist or a counsellor.

3. If you find that the professional help and advice you are given is not working for you, try one of the voluntary organizations mentioned in the back of the book. Don't be afraid to shop around for the right solution to your particular problem. If you find the professionals resistant to the idea of your having an illness in the first place, take the advice of the Association for Post-Natal Illness (page 113) and get hold of some literature to show to them.

4. Don't suffer in silence and alone.

CHAPTER NINE

Where to find help

Clare Delpech gave birth to her third baby in 1979 after having no problems with her first two children. Her post-natal depression went undiagnosed for a long time, mainly she feels, because she did not feel depressed, she felt physically ill. It must be stressed that not everyone has the same experience or symptoms as Clare. At one point her GP asked her if she felt depressed, but she told him no, she just felt terribly ill.

Clare's story

He was born in January, and I didn't feel well right from the beginning. Then a couple of months after the birth I had to have several minor operations in a row. I felt no better after those and in fact, began to feel worse and worse and less and less capable of looking after the baby, let alone the rest of the family. Then in May I began to feel suicidal. I'd been in hospital, and being separated from the baby and the rest of the family made matters worse. When I came out of hospital I just rotted at home for six weeks. The problem seemed to be physical and in desperation one day I phoned up my obstetrician because I felt so ill. I spoke to his secretary who I know quite well and told her what the symptoms were and she said 'I'm sure you have post-natal depression' and she went on to describe how it was. She told me she'd been terribly ill with it herself and she was sure that's what the matter was. She spoke to the obstetrician and it was decided that I needed to see the psychiatrist at the hospital where I had the baby. She was a tremendous woman, absolutely lovely. PND was one of her major interests and she helped me a lot.

By that time I was scarcely able to go out of the house. I was unable to cope with the baby. My mother was staying with us looking after the baby and she hired a nanny to look after the two older ones. If I hadn't had this help, they would have had to take the children into care I was in such a state.

When I saw the psychiatrist, she said, 'Yes, it's run-of-the-mill PND and I'm sure that with the right medication you'll soon be better'. Finding the right anti-depressant for me was not easy, but once we'd got that sorted out in a very few weeks, I was much better and starting to function again. By September I was well enough to take my eldest daughter to school on her first day, which would have been unheard of only a couple of months before that.

I was a biochemist by training, and I had to find out more about this thing. Because of my job, I knew some of the people at the hospital (Queen Charlotte's, the famous London maternity hospital) and one professor in particular was very helpful. He told me there was nothing for people who become ill with this and that it was very badly publicized. I made no secret of the fact that I was quite ill at the time, but I determined to do something about this situation and he helped me to start the Association for Post-natal Illness (page 112) and to get it going.

While I was ill it helped me a lot to talk to the obstetrician's secretary. She seemed to be the only person who knew what it was like. People used to gasp and shudder when you talked about the symptoms. I remember she described it for me once. What happens when you go into a shop, for instance, is that you look round the shelves and everything is just a blur. You stand there in a fog totally unable to do anything or decide anything. And then you panic. That to me was a wonderful description of having the illness. There are times when you are so detached from what's going on around you that you don't know where you are and you wonder 'how can I get back?' It's appalling that mothers in that condition are left alone to look after tiny children when they really aren't capable.

It really is a serious illness. The vast majority of people don't realize how ill people can become. Women commit suicide they are so desperate and we hear about them regularly. Knowing that you can kill yourself somehow keeps you going because life is such hell. Some women in that situation actually do it. It's no cry for help, there's no fudging, they want to kill themselves.

I was very lucky. My family really took care of me. They made sure somebody was with me all the time. My mother would go off duty when my husband came in the door from work. I feel very sorry for husbands in this situation. They have a perfectly happy wife who has a baby and appears to fall apart. It's terrible to watch the slow decline from a nice person to be with into a hopeless, neurotic, tearful wreck. My husband is a kind and sympathetic man and he was absolutely convinced that I would recover. I wouldn't have been like that to him, I'm sure. It's terribly hard to understand that this is an illness, that you will get better. Once men realize that they will have their wives back again and that it isn't her fault, then things are better for everyone involved.

How the Association for Post-natal Illness works

The Association for Post-natal Illness is involved in four areas of work: information and education, research into causes and treatments of the illness and, possibly most important of all, support for victims of the illness. There is a membership of over 3000 people and in the years since it started, over 1000 mothers have been supported and are now recovered from the illness. This work is done by an army of between 650 and 700 volunteers from around the country.

Clare Delpech is very aware that having lay people as volunteers can lead to problems and there are golden rules which the association always follows. First of all, they never diagnose. 'This is a trap which voluntary organizations have a tendency to fall into,' says Clare Delpech, 'but we never, ever do that.' This is why the association stresses its professional links and has a medical committee on which sit some of the top names in obstetrics and psychiatry in the field of post-natal depression.

'We are dealing with women who are extremely ill,' says Delpech. 'Trying to do good isn't enough. We have to be really sure we aren't doing any harm. It is a very difficult thing to diagnose. Most people tend to go to the doctor complaining of one symptom and very often doctors just don't have the time to go into things more deeply.'

The condition is underestimated, she feels, because women are still walking, talking and look reasonably normal. The only physical sign is a certain pallor but of course that is difficult to spot and could also be a pointer to a host of other conditions. Delpech says that a 'rash of purple spots would be much better' for everyone concerned. She is keen to emphasize that it is a medical condition following childbirth, not just a psychiatric problem. It is the major maternal illness, it is a killer and one that should not be ignored. She had hoped, she said, that when she started the association in the late 1970s it would no longer be necessary after 10 years. But the work goes on.

Counselling acts as a lifeline for many sick mothers, and Delpech is convinced that it has prevented many deaths. She is full of praise for volunteers, because it is, she says, quite unlike being a Samaritan, for instance, because the volunteers never go off duty and are often called right through the night by women at the height of their illness. It is a question of changing attitudes both among the medical profession and the public.

To this end the association recommends that the first thing a woman who thinks she is suffering from PND should do is to send for some literature. It is their experience that actually having something in print helps not only the victim but the people around her. It can be particularly helpful for those who have not had sympathy and understanding and whose relatives have doubted them. Sufferers are advised to give the information to their families and to their doctor if necessary. 'To a GP, you can say this is what I've got, please treat me. And on several occasions partners have told us that it made all the difference to see it in black and white. It has worked and it has changed attitudes.'

The association also has a few basic suggestions to help women who are suffering to simply get through the day. They are anxious to emphasize that there are no instant cures, that it will take time, but also, on the positive side, to emphasize that women will recover.

An Association for Post-natal Illness check list of self-help

1. Work out which part of the day is the worst for you and plan to do the chores which you have to get through at the other end of the day. This means that you won't have to struggle on through the worst patch, and also that you will at least be able to achieve something. Some women who are able and want to go back to work, are often helped by the structure and rewards of a job.

2. Most women suffering from PND find that they lose their appetite. But eating is very important, because if the blood sugar level drops, that too can affect how you feel. So eating something sweet little and often is recommended if you are going through a stage when you really cannot face a proper meal. A piece of fruit, or a couple of teaspoons of honey every couple of hours will help keep your glucose levels up and may well keep you off rock bottom when you're feeling down.

3. Most sufferers have sleep problems at some time or another. Either they wake up suddenly after a terrible nightmare, or they wake regularly and are unable to get back to sleep. The way to approach this problem is first of all to stop worrying about not sleeping. Just lying in bed is resting and while you may not feel all that much better for it, it is still doing some good. Some women begin to panic about not sleeping, but once you've got over these worries about it, you will find it much easier to sleep. It's an idea to make up a thermos so that you can have a warm drink sitting up in bed. If you find yourself lying there worrying, do something to take your mind off it, such as reading or knitting or sewing, something you enjoy. The important thing to remember is not to fret and this in itself takes the pressure off.

4. Your family must help you out by reducing the stress of everyday life which you find so difficult to bear. If there are any problems, they must be prepared to help you out and cope with them on your behalf. If, for example, you have to move house during this time, you cannot be counted on

to cope with it at all. They must organize it for you. They must realize and accept that PND is a serious illness and you are handicapped because of it.

5. Many women find that they suffer from agoraphobia and cannot bear to leave the security of their own homes. Others find that they cannot bear to be at home and so try to get out all the time. While psychiatrists might argue that you should not let a phobia have its way, it must be remembered that this is a symptom of your illness and not an illness in itself. Lots of women have phobias about what appears on television, becoming very frightened by news programmes for instance. Or they cannot bear to read sad stories in the newspapers. It is unpleasant and very distressing for the person who is suffering from this irrational fear, as well as those around her who witness it. Clare Delpech remembers her own phobia which concerned a balcony leading from her bedroom through a door. Once her husband had tied up the door with a piece of rope, convincing her that the door could not fly open at any time, she suddenly felt safe. It was a great relief and eventually after a couple of months when she was feeling better, the rope was untied and she felt fine. She urges relatives who find themselves in this situation to consider getting rid of the television, or cancelling the newspapers for a while until the worry has subsided. After all, it is only a temporary measure.

6. Women who are working face special problems. Many push themselves to get back to work as quickly as possible. But this should be avoided as this sort of stress faced too soon may only make things worse. However important the job may seem, you must face the fact that you cannot work if you are ill. You must wait until you feel ready to cope with this particular pressure.

A PND postscript

As a final idea if you are suffering from post-natal depression and you feel you have no one to talk to, it sometimes helps to write things down. You could try keeping a diary. It might help clarify your thoughts and also, as you begin to feel better, it will help you to see that the good days are beginning to outnumber the bad days.

You might also like to try and answer for yourself the same questions I asked the women I spoke to during the writing of this book.

1. How was your pregnancy? Was it normal and did you enjoy it?

2. How was the birth? On balance would you say it was a good experience?

3. Did you breastfeed or bottlefeed your baby and how did you settle down together?

4. Did you suffer the 'blues'?

5. Did you feel you got a sympathetic response from hospital staff, midwives and family to that experience?

6. Did you get depressed after your first or subsequent pregnancies?

7. Have you ever suffered from depression before?

8. Have any other close relatives suffered from depression or anyone else in your family, e.g. mother, sister, ever suffered from post-natal depression?

9. What sort of support did you get from your family, your doctor, midwife, health visitor, friends?

10. Did you realize you were suffering from depression?

11. Who first suggested you might be suffering from post-natal depression?

12. What symptoms did you have and how long did they last?

13. Were health professionals, such as your doctor or midwife supportive?

14. Did anyone tell you about post-natal depression when you were pregnant?

15. Did you know anyone else who was depressed?

16. Was your baby happy and contented or do you feel he/she cried a lot and was difficult to satisfy?

17. Did you enjoy your baby during those early weeks?

18. Did your depression affect your relationship with your partner, your baby, your family?

19. Who did you find the most helpful and supportive during your illness?

20. What professional help or treatment did you receive?

21. Do you think you are fully recovered?

22. Did the experience put you off having other children?

23. How did you cope?

24. Did you have a job before the baby and did you go back to work afterwards?

25. Do you think you had any idea what motherhood would be like?

26. What advice would you give to other sufferers?

27. Who helped you most?

28. Do you think your child has suffered in any way because of your illness?

29. Do you think those around you understand how you were feeling?

30. Would it have helped you to talk to someone who had also suffered from this illness?

International help and support groups

Australia

The Nursing Mothers' Association of Australia have branches in most states and can often help with advice and counselling. They are a fairly informal organization and you can find your nearest branch in the local telephone directory under the heading 'Nursing Mothers'. The National Headquarters is at P.O. Box 231, 5 Glendale Road, Nunawading, Victoria 3131. A counselling service is available on (3) 878 3304. The headquarters' telephone number is (3) 877 5011.

PaNDa — Post- and Ante-Natal Depression Association. A support and information group, started in 1983, for women who experience PND and their families. It is run by a management committee of women who have personal experience of PND and there is a network of 20 groups throughout Victoria. PaNDa offers twice-monthly newsletters which are available nationally and the group organizes four information nights each year which are filmed and then made available to the public. The organization also has an information package which contains the latest information about PND and its treatments and any news about research findings. There is a country-wide telephone support system and various groups hold regular get-togethers.

There is also a PND Clinic at the Royal Women's Hospital, Gratan St Carlton, Melbourne and a Post-Natal Disorder Clinic and Mother-Baby Unit at the Mercy Maternity Hospital, Bundoora. For more information write to PaNDa at 14 Lillimur Road, Ormond, Victoria 3163.

La Leche League offers information and support for women who want to know more about breastfeeding. Their members are trained counsellors, all of whom are mothers who have themselves breastfed. The League also offers a local support group and telephone service for mothers who need help.

La Leche League Australia
c/o Pinky McKay
8 Gateshed Drive
Wantirna
Victoria 3182
(3) 221 1997

New Zealand

La Leche League of New Zealand
PO Box 13-383
Wellington 4
(24) 785 213

USA

In America, there are various organizations to help mothers who feel they are having problems. One such is Postpartum Education for Parents (PEP), P.O. Box 6154, Santa Barbara, California 93160. It was started in the 1970s by three professional women who all encountered problems as first-time mothers. They offer a 24-hour telephone service and various support groups for mothers. It is not designed primarily for mothers suffering from post-natal depression, but the group can offer support to mothers with problems.

Another similar group is MELD (Minnesota Early Learning Design) which was originally set up in Minneapolis. It now has almost 50 groups all over the USA. It divides its work into several areas, depending on a child's development and age. There are five main areas: child development, child guidance, health, family management, and personal growth. The organization works by setting up groups where parents can support each other with the help of a facilitator. For more information write to MELD, 123 East Grand Street, Minneapolis, Minnesota 55403.

The Mothers' Centre group is organized along similar lines to the above, but usually deals only with mothers. There are a number of these groups in New York State. Contact the Mothers' Centre Development Project, 129 Jackson Street, Hempstead, New York, NY 11550.

La Leche League International
PO Box 1209
Franklin Park
Chicago
Illinois 6031-8209
(708) 455 7730

Marcé Society
Dr Michael O'Hara
Department of Psychology
University of Iowa
Iowa 52242

Canada

The Pacific Post Partum Support Society
888 Burrard Street
Vancouver
BC V6Z 1X9

La Leche League Canada
493 Main Street
Winchester
Ontario K0C 2K0
(613) 774 2850

Secretariat Générale de la Leche League
Case postale 874
Ville St Laurent
Quebec H4L 4W3
(514) 327 6714

UK

In Britain, there are a number of organizations which offer help and support for families with difficulties, or for those who simply want information. When writing, please enclose a stamped, self-addressed envelope.

The Association for Post-Natal Illness
7 Gowan Avenue
Fulham
London SW6 6RH
071-731 4867

Birthright
27 Sussex Place
Regent's Park
London NW1 4SP
071-262 5337

MAMA, the Meet-A-Mum Association, has a network of self-help groups all over the country for mothers of small children. There are coffee mornings, visits, lectures and the group can also help mums to find friends and has a number of contacts who can help via the telephone with common problems associated with having babies: depression, guilt, medical problems, loneliness, etc.

MAMA
c/o Mrs Valerie Dallinger
5 Westbury Gardens
Luton LU2 7DW
(0582) 422253

The National Childbirth Trust provides ante-natal classes for pregnant women and continues with support after the birth of the baby, including sympathetic help with post-natal problems such as depression. They run a post-natal network which has branches all over the country.

The National Childbirth Trust
Alexandra House
Oldham Terrace
Acton
London W3 6NH
081-992 8637

Mother and Baby magazine runs a contact page called 'In Touch' for lonely mums which can be particularly helpful if you've just moved house. You can buy it at any newsagents.

CRY-SIS is an organization for parents who find it difficult to cope with their baby's continual crying. Volunteers who have experience of the problem offer support and practical help.

BM CRY-SIS
London WC1N 3XX
071-404 5011

OPUS (Organization for Parents Under Stress)
106 Godstone Road
Whyteleafe
Surrey CR3 0EB
081-645 0469

Pre-School Playgroups Association
Alford House
Aveline Street
London SE11 5DH
071-582 8871

Relate, formerly the National Marriage Guidance Council. See your local directory for the nearest branch, or contact headquarters.

Herbert Gray College
Little Church Street
Rugby
Warwickshire CV21 3AP
(0788) 73241

AIMS (Association for Improvements in Maternity Services)
The Secretary
163 Liverpool Road
London N1 0RF
071-491 2772

The Maternity Alliance
15 Britannia Street
London WC1X 9JP
071-837 1265

La Leche League of Great Britain
BM 3424
London WC1N 3XX
071-242 1278

MIND, the National Association for Mental Health
22 Harley Street
London W1N 2ED
071-637 0741

The National Council for One-Parent Families
255 Kentish Town Road
London NW5 2LX
071-267 1361

NSPCC, the National Society for the Prevention of Cruelty to
Children
67 Saffron Hill
London EC1N 8RS
071-242 1626, or see your local directory for local numbers.
Offer confidential and sympathetic support for mothers and
publish *Putting Children First, A Guide for Parents of 0-5 year
olds.*

SANDS, the Stillbirth and Neonatal Death Society
Argyle House
29-31 Euston Road
London NW1 3SD
071-833 2851

The Miscarriage Association
11 Bank Street
Ossett
W. Yorkshire
(092) 485 515

The Twins and Multiple Births Association
Katy Gow
1 Victoria Place
King's Park
Stirling SK 3QX
(0786) 72080

Marcé Society
Dr Beth Alder
Department of Community Studies
Queen Margaret College
Clerwood Terrace
Edinburgh EH12 8TS
Professional society with the aim of improving the under-
standing and prevention of mental illness relating to
childbearing. Publish annual bulletin for members and
updated reading list on the subject of PND.

Recommended reading for new mothers

The Association for Post-Natal Illness has a number of leaflets
on post-natal depression, write to them at the address above.

*Depression after Childbirth: How to recognize and treat
postnatal illness,* Dr Katharina Dalton, Oxford University
Press.

*The New Mother Syndrome: Coping with pre-natal stress and
depression,* Carol Dix, Unwin Paperbacks.

Postnatal Depression, Vivienne Welburn, Fontana Paperbacks.

Postnatal Depression: A guide for health professionals, John L. Cox, Churchill Livingstone.

Comfort for Depression, Janet Horwood, Sheldon Press.

Primal Health: A blueprint for our survival, Michel Odent, Century.

How to Have a Baby and Stay Sane, Virginia Ironside, Unwin Hyman.

Understanding Mental Health, Angelina Gibbs, a Which? book.

Kitchen Sink, or Swim? Women in the eighties — the choices, Deidre Sanders with Jane Reed, Pelican.

New Mothers at Work: Employment and childcare, Julia Brannen and Peter Moss, Unwin Paperbacks.

The Good Nanny Guide, Charlotte Breese and Hilaire Gomer, Century.

Babyshock — A mother's first five years, Dr John Cobb, Arrow Paperbacks.

Motherhood and Mental Illness, vol II, R. Kumar and I.F. Brockington (eds), Wright.

Index